BODYWEIGHT
STRENGTH TRAINING
ANATOMY

Bret Contreras

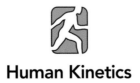

Human Kinetics

Library of Congress Cataloging-in-Publication Data

Contreras, Bret, 1976-
  Bodyweight strength training anatomy / Bret Contreras.
    pages cm
1. Bodybuilding--Training. 2. Muscle strength. I. Title.
  GV546.5.C655 2013
  613.7'13--dc23

                                                2013013580

  ISBN: 978-1-4504-2929-0 (print)

Acquisitions Editor: Tom Heine; **Developmental Editor:** Cynthia McEntire; **Assistant Editor:** Elizabeth Evans; **Copyeditor:** Annette Pierce; **Graphic Designer:** Fred Starbird; **Graphic Artist:** Kim McFarland; **Cover Designer:** Keith Blomberg; **Photographer (for cover and interior illustration references):** Neil Bernstein; **Visual Production Assistant:** Joyce Brumfield; **Art Manager:** Kelly Hendren; **Associate Art Manager:** Alan L. Wilborn; **Illustrator (cover and interior):** Jen Gibas; **Printer:** Versa Press

Printed in the United States of America   20 19 18 17 16 15 14 13 12 11

The paper in this book is certified under a sustainable forestry program.

Human Kinetics
P.O. Box 5076
Champaign, IL 61825-5076
Website: www.HumanKinetics.com

In the United States, email info@hkusa.com or call 800-747-4457.
In Canada, email info@hkcanada.com.
In the United Kingdom/Europe, email hk@hkeurope.com.

For information about Human Kinetics' coverage in other areas of the world, please visit our website: **www.HumanKinetics.com**

E5716

BODYWEIGHT
STRENGTH TRAINING
ANATOMY

CONTENTS

PREFACE

Because you're reading this book, I think it's safe to say that you're interested in learning how to build strength and fitness through bodyweight training. If so, that's great! You've come to the right place.

Over the past 20 years, I've never taken more than a few days off from strength training. Although I've trained in hundreds of amazing gyms, studios, and facilities, on many occasions I've had to make do with what I had in my house, apartment, or hotel room. When I first started training with weights at the age of 15, I didn't know what I was doing. I remember feeling awkward, uncomfortable, and uncoordinated with many of the exercises. As a matter of fact, I avoided most multijoint exercises because I didn't feel them working the way I felt isolation exercises working. Looking back, I realize that I was a skinny weakling who possessed extremely inferior levels of core stability, single-leg stability, and motor control. I simply wandered around aimlessly without a plan, moving randomly from one exercise to another.

At first, I couldn't perform push-ups so I didn't bother trying them. In fact, I couldn't perform a chin-up, dip, or inverted row, either. I suspect that had I attempted a bodyweight full squat my back would have rounded and my knees would have caved in (the melting-candle syndrome) because my glutes were incredibly weak and I had no knowledge of proper form. It took me five years to be able to perform a bodyweight chin-up and dip.

I've spent the past 20 years learning as much as I can possibly learn about the human body as it pertains to strength and conditioning. Had I known then what I know now, I could have accelerated my results by several years by sticking to a proper exercise progression system and program template. I venture to guess that I could have been performing chin-ups and dips within my first year of training had I possessed a sound understanding of form, exercise progression, and program design. I want to go back in time to help my younger, confused (but determined) self. I wish that the current me could mentor the former me and teach him the ropes.

Flash forward 20 years. I feel great, my joint health is outstanding, my strength levels are highly advanced, and my muscle control is superior. I'm now able to achieve an amazing workout using just my own body weight and simple household furniture. I lean my back on couches in order to work my glutes. I hang on to tables and chairs to work my back and legs. And all I need is the ground to work my chest, shoulders, legs, and core.

I believe that all strength trainees should master their own body weight as a form of resistance before moving on to free weights and other training systems. Bodyweight exercises lay the foundation for future training success, and correct performance requires a precise blend of mobility, stability, and motor control. As you make progress and gain strength, it is possible to continue to push yourself through bodyweight training so you continue to challenge the muscles and increase your athleticism. But you need to learn the exercises and have a road map to help get you there.

Bodyweight Strength Training Anatomy was written for several categories of people:

- Beginners who need to learn the basics of bodyweight training. Everyone knows about push-ups and squats, but not everyone knows about hip thrusts, RKC planks, and inverted rows. These exercises should be staples of every strength enthusiast's routine.

- Folks who want to be in great shape but don't like attending gyms. If this describes you, then rest assured that you will always be able to receive an amazing workout no matter where you are.

- Fit exercisers who do a lot of traveling. Sure it's nice to have access to hundreds of thousands of dollars of strength training equipment, but if you're frequently on the road then you know that this option is not always feasible.

- All strength training enthusiasts. Regardless of whether you're a weekend warrior, an athlete, a lifter, a coach, a trainer, or a therapist, if your line of work involves fitness then you need to understand bodyweight strength training. Strength training enthusiasts may have specific fitness goals, such as improving functional strength, gaining muscle, losing fat, or improving posture, and bodyweight training will help each of these people achieve those goals.

Here is how I lay out the book. Chapter 1 introduces bodyweight training. Chapters 2 through 9 discuss functional anatomy and its role in sports and aesthetics and lay out the best bodyweight exercises for these muscle groups: arms, neck and shoulders, chest, core, back, thighs, glutes, and calves. In chapter 10, I go over whole-body exercises and explain their purpose. Finally, in chapter 11, the most important chapter of all, I teach you the basics of program design and provide several sample templates for you to follow. *Bodyweight Strength Training Anatomy* features drawings, instructions, and descriptions of approximately 150 exercises for you to reference. As you progress in strength, you'll be able to advance from easier to more difficult exercise variations, and I include a rating system to help you determine the level of difficulty of each exercise.

Beginner

Intermediate

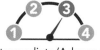
Intermediate/Advanced

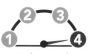
Advanced

Unique to *Bodyweight Strength Training Anatomy* are detailed pictures to help you identify the muscle groups and muscle parts that are stressed during an exercise. Research has shown that it is possible to target a particular area of a muscle, but in order to do so it is essential to be aware of the muscle in order to target that region while training. Primary and secondary muscles featured in each exercise are color coded within the anatomical illustrations that accompany the exercises to help you develop your mind–muscle connection.

☐ Primary muscles   ☐ Secondary muscles

After reading *Bodyweight Strength Training Anatomy,* you'll possess a sound understanding of the muscle groups within the human body and will know plenty of exercises that train each movement pattern and muscle. You will know how to properly perform bodyweight exercises that are critical to future improvements. You will understand where to start and how to progress so you can develop proper flexibility and strength to keep advancing over time. You will know the important roles that core stability and gluteal strength play in fundamental movement, and you'll understand how to design effective programs based on your uniqueness and preferences. Finally, you'll dramatically increase your appreciation of bodyweight training, the most convenient form of strength training.

ACKNOWLEDGMENTS

I would like to thank my good friend Brad Schoenfeld. Not only did he recommend me to Human Kinetics, but he also provided much-needed expertise as I worked my way through the publication of my first book. I would also like to thank my family for always being so supportive.

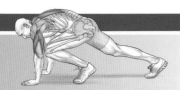

chapter 1

THE BODYWEIGHT CHALLENGE

Numerous books have been written on training with one's body weight. Most include a compendium of exercises common to bodyweight training. However, a large collection of exercises is only part of the package. The results you achieve depend on a variety of factors, and it's important that you perform the best exercise variations and adhere to a well-balanced routine.

Although I've been resistance training for 20 years, I've spent the past decade delving into the world of strength and conditioning. I've learned from the world's best coaches, biomechanists, physical therapists, and researchers. So I speak from experience in stating that when you've been in the game for long enough, you can simply glance at a program and know right away whether the program is efficient and will deliver optimal results.

When it comes to program design, I trust strength coaches over just about anyone. Not only do they have a vested interest in optimizing their athletes' strength, power, and conditioning, but they also must consider the crucial issues of joint health and longevity. As such, their job is to put together sound programs that will ensure progression while preventing dysfunctional adaptations.

PUSHING AND PULLING

It's important to understand that bodyweight training is highly skewed toward pushing over pulling. Because of the wonders of gravity, all it takes to get a great pressing workout is to sink your body toward the ground and then push your body upward. Think of squats, lunges, push-ups, and handstand push-ups. These are great pressing movements that you should definitely be performing. But what about pulling movements? You can't grip the ground and pull yourself anywhere.

Bodyweight pulling exercises require the use of a pull-up bar, suspension system, or sturdy pieces of furniture if the other equipment is unavailable. You can maneuver your body around the furniture in order to strengthen the pulling muscles that provide structural balance to your body and counteract the postural adaptations imposed by the pressing movements.

Nearly all of the at-home bodyweight programs I've seen are in fact slanted toward pressing movements. Although these pressing exercises are highly effective, programs must devote equal attention to exercise order as well as the number

Chin-Up Bars and Suspension Systems

You may find it more comfortable to perform pull-up and row variations from an actual chin-up bar and suspension system instead of a solid and sturdy door, rafter, or table. Consider making your own chin-up bar or inverted row station or purchasing one. These days you can find plenty of models, such as the Iron Gym or the TRX, which you simply install above a doorframe. Doing so will allow you to perform the movements using different grips with more natural movement.

of exercises, sets, and repetitions dedicated to pulling movements. Otherwise structural imbalances result. Quadriceps dominance and knee pain, rounded shoulders and shoulder pain, and anterior (forward) pelvic tilt and lower-back pain are just some of the negative effects that someone could experience after following a poorly designed program.

I took on the challenge of writing this book for two reasons. First, a high-quality bodyweight training book centered on proper exercise selection and balanced program design was sorely needed in the industry. Second, I'm passionate about bodyweight training. I don't believe that anyone else has devoted as much consideration to bodyweight exercises for the muscles on the back of the body. As noted, it's easy to work the muscles on the front of the body with bodyweight training because these are the pushing muscles. But an athletic and fit person requires strong muscles on the back of the body as well, and the bodyweight pulling exercises that work these muscles aren't so straightforward. They require creativity.

THE BODYWEIGHT ADVANTAGE

Many folks absolutely love the prospect of being able to train efficiently in the convenience of their own home. Most fitness enthusiasts have gym memberships and have become highly dependent on machines and free weights to work their muscles. While I'm a huge proponent of using all types of resistance, bodyweight training is without a doubt the most convenient type of resistance. All you need is your own physical being, and you'll never be without equipment or a facility and you'll never need a spotter. In other words, if you learn to use your body as a barbell then you'll always have the ability to obtain a great workout. You can gain tremendous functional fitness in terms of strength, power, balance, and endurance from progressive bodyweight training, and recent research shows that you can enhance your flexibility to the same or even a greater degree through resistance training than from a stretching routine.

I like to watch all types of athletes train. As a strength coach I've watched thousands of athletes lift weights. Two types of athletes have always stood out to me in terms of superior muscular control: gymnasts and bodybuilders. In awe, I watch the gymnast on the rings or the pommel horse maneuvering his body around the apparatus with precision. I watch the bodybuilder contract his or her muscles against the resistance with total concentration. When training with body weight, you want to learn from these athletes and develop a tremendous mind–muscle connection, which will allow you to achieve an amazing workout anywhere you go.

In this book I will teach you the best bodyweight exercises and show you the most effective way to combine them into cohesive programs consistent with your fitness goals. You will learn how to progress from the simplest variations to the most complicated and advanced bodyweight exercises. You will learn to use your abdominals and gluteals to lock your torso into position and create a stiff pillar of support while you move your limbs. You will become lean, limber, and athletic. Push-ups and pull-ups won't intimidate you. Your glutes will function like never before, and the confidence you gain from this program will shine through in every aspect of your life.

You will never fear having subpar training sessions when you go on vacation because you'll be able to perform an effective workout from the comfort of your hotel room. You'll realize that you don't need barbells, dumbbells, or elastic resistance bands. With sound knowledge of the biomechanics of bodyweight training, you can learn to create just as much force in the muscles as if performing heavy resistance training.

Better yet, you'll save thousands on gym membership fees without compromising the quality of your workout. You can use these savings to make healthier food choices so you can realize even better results from your training. All in the comfort of your own home!

I was recently asked whether or not I believed that I could maintain my muscularity and fitness solely by performing bodyweight exercises. Without hesitation I answered, "Yes." As you progress to more difficult variations and increase the number of repetitions you perform with the various exercises, you

Safety First!

Although I will teach you how to perform many exercises using standard furniture, I don't want you to get injured if a chair slides or a door comes off its hinges. Remember that standard fitness equipment such as chin-up bars and weight benches are viable options as well. If you do choose to use furniture, I emphatically remind you that every piece of furniture you use when training must be secure, stable, and strong. Placing the furniture against a wall or on top of a sturdy rug will prevent it from sliding around. Wedging a book beneath an open door will provide extra support. If there is a risk you might slip and fall, perform the exercise over a soft surface such as carpeting or turf. Test the safety of your setup with one or two repetitions before beginning your full workout. If a particular setup seems unbalanced or insecure, switch to a different exercise or explore a safer alternative.

will continuously challenge your neuromuscular system. Your body will respond by synthesizing more protein and laying down more muscle tissue. In essence, your body adapts by building a bigger engine. Recent studies have shown that high repetitions can provide a potent muscle-building stimulus, more so than most experts imagined. I'm glad you've decided to take the bodyweight challenge and learn how to manipulate your body to achieve a world-class workout. I'm glad that you've decided to no longer be a slave to the gym. Now the world is your gym and you are the resistance.

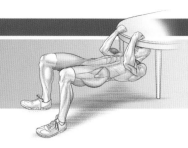

ARMS

Talk to any teenage boy who is new to strength training and chances are the first thing he'll ask you about is arm training. Among men, well-developed biceps and triceps are likely the most coveted muscles in the body. This makes perfect sense. They're the least covered major muscles of the body. Shirts, pants, shorts, and socks conceal most of the torso and legs, but usually the arms are right out in the open in plain view for everyone to see.

You'll be hard-pressed to find muscles that are flexed more often in bathrooms across the world than the arms, because at any given point probably thousands of guys are striking double biceps poses in front of their mirrors. When you have string bean arms, you'll do just about anything to fill out your shirtsleeves with a muscular set of guns. While the biceps seem to get all the glory, the appearance of the arms requires proper development of the triceps on the back of the arms as well.

Arm exercises aren't just for men. They're important for women, too. First lady Michelle Obama created a media buzz with her muscular, toned arms. Talk to a soon-to-be bride or bridesmaid who will sport a strapless dress and she'll let you know how much she covets well-defined arm muscles. Many women are insecure about the appearance of their triceps in particular and seek to firm the area by increasing muscle development through triceps-strengthening exercises.

MUSCLES OF THE ARMS

To better understand how to best target the arm musculature, let's first delve into basic anatomy. On the front of the upper arms, you have the elbow flexors. Elbow flexion is moving the wrist toward the shoulder by bending the arm. The primary elbow flexors are the biceps brachii, which are actually composed of two heads, a long head and a short head (figure 2.1). Other elbow flexors you should know about are the brachialis and brachioradialis. These muscles contribute to movement in varying degrees depending on how the elbow flexion exercise is performed. In general, the biceps brachii is worked most with a supinated (palms-up) grip, the brachioradialis with a neutral grip (palms facing each other), and the brachialis with a pronated (palms-down) grip. This is because of the leverage of each muscle at various positions and ranges of motions.

The back of the upper arm is composed of the elbow extensors. Elbow extension is moving the wrist away from the shoulder by straightening the arm to form a solid line from shoulder to wrist. The primary elbow extensors consist of the

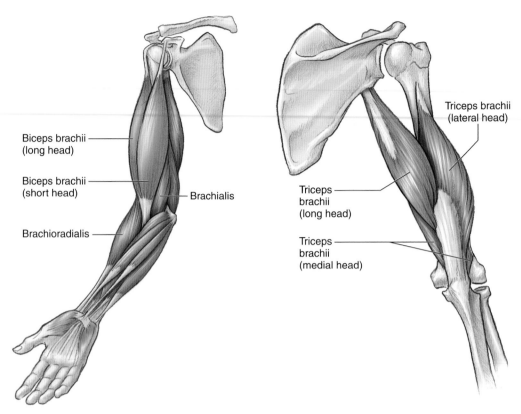

Figure 2.1   Biceps brachii, brachialis, and brachioradialis.

Figure 2.2   Triceps brachii.

three individual heads of the triceps brachii—the long head, medial head, and lateral head (figure 2.2).

The arms are important in various athletic pursuits. The elbow extensors contract forcefully when swinging a baseball bat or golf club, when stiff-arming or pushing an opponent forward in American football, when going for a spike in volleyball, or when throwing a ball overhead in baseball or American football. These muscles are heavily involved in throwing a chest pass in basketball or a jab or right cross in boxing or heaving a shot put in track and field.

The elbow flexors transfer energy when swinging a racket in tennis or a hook in boxing. They're relied on when clinching or attempting or avoiding arm-bar submissions in mixed martial arts, when tackling an opponent in American football, and when pulling the body up in rock climbing. In addition, they're involved in carrying heavy objects out in front of the body in strongman events and in the sport of rowing.

EXERCISING THE ARMS

The arms are worked heavily during upper-body exercises that involve the movement of two or more joints at a time. All types of pull-up and rowing motions will sufficiently work the elbow flexors, and all types of push-up and dipping motions will sufficiently work the elbow extensors. For this reason, every time you train your chest, shoulders, and back you'll necessarily be working your arms.

The involvement of the arm musculature during multijoint movements is particularly important from a bodyweight training perspective. It's easy to isolate the arm muscles when using free weights or cables. Simply grab a weighted implement and flex or extend the elbows. Things become more complicated, however, when trying to use your body as a barbell. It's difficult to manipulate the body around the elbow joints. This isn't to say that it's not a good idea to try to target the arms with single-joint movements. But it is critical to understand that multijoint movements are the most productive in terms of total muscular output.

When performing arm exercises, concentrate on squeezing the intended muscles and don't allow other muscles to do the job. Before heavy sets of elbow flexion exercises, Arnold Schwarzenegger used to envision his biceps growing as big as mountains. Focus on feeling the arm muscles contracting in order to create the desired movement. Bodybuilders call this a mind–muscle connection, and it takes time to sufficiently develop these neuromuscular pathways. Training for sport and functional purposes is more about training movements; whereas training for physique and aesthetic purposes is more about training muscles. For this reason, think about arm training as contracting your muscles against resistance. This will help you put maximal stress on the intended muscles.

Although the forearms are indeed part of the arms, they will be worked during gripping movements, including pull-ups and rowing motions, while training the back musculature. (See chapter 6.)

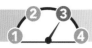

ARMS

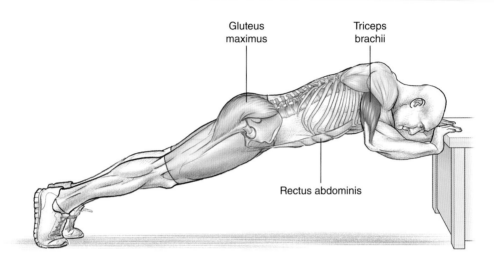

Gluteus maximus

Triceps brachii

Rectus abdominis

Safety Tip > Choose a stable, sturdy table, or chair.

Execution

1. Place your hands on the corner of a table or seat of a chair and back into proper position.
2. Keeping your body in a straight line with straight legs, straight arms, weight on the toes, and the abdominals and glutes braced, lower your body by bending the elbows.
3. Raise the body by using the triceps to extend the elbows.

Muscles Involved

Primary: Triceps brachii

Secondary: Rectus abdominis, gluteus maximus

Exercise Notes

The triceps extension is one of the rare exercises that truly targets the triceps musculature. This is because the body revolves around the elbow joint with nearly pure elbow extension. Get into a strong position by planting firmly into the ground and squeezing the abdominals and glutes to maintain a solid straight line from head to toe. Do not lose this position during the exercise. Losing this position by sagging at the hips is not only unathletic but is also potentially harmful to the low back. Don't allow the shoulder joint to move much and try to keep most of the movement around the elbows. Use the triceps musculature to raise and lower the body.

You can modulate the difficulty of this exercise by adjusting the chair or table height. To make the exercise easier, use a taller chair or table. Conversely, to make the exercise more difficult, use a shorter chair or table.

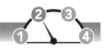

‹ VARIATION ›

Short-Lever Triceps Extension

People who find this movement challenging may shorten the lever by performing the movement from the knees, thereby reducing the total percentage of body weight being lifted. Use a sturdy chair or coffee table for this exercise; a standard table is too high.

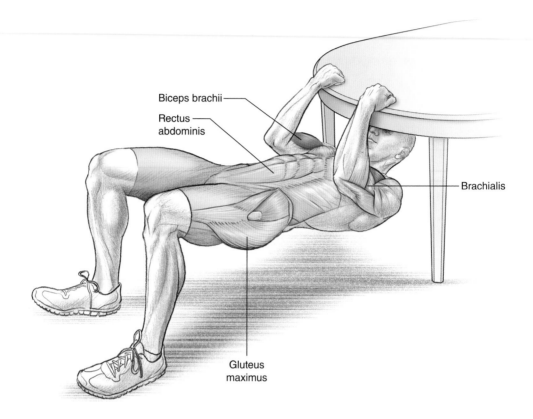

Biceps brachii
Rectus abdominis
Brachialis
Gluteus maximus

Safety Tip Choose a sturdy table or chair. Perform the exercise over a soft surface such as carpeting.

Execution

1. Lying on your back, set up under a sturdy table or tall chair with your hands grasping the outer edges, palms facing each other.

2. With your torso and legs in a straight line, neck in neutral position, knees bent at 90 degrees, weight on the heels, and the abdominals and glutes braced, raise your body by bending the elbows. (When the neck is in neutral position, the head and neck remain in their natural positions and are not tilted up or back.)

3. Lower to starting position under control, moving mostly at the elbows and not the shoulders.

Muscles Involved

Primary: Biceps brachii

Secondary: Brachialis, rectus abdominis, gluteus maximus

Exercise Notes

The short-lever inverted curl is one of the only pure biceps exercises. Most of the other biceps movements heavily involve the muscles of the back. Make sure you squeeze the core muscles including the glutes in order to keep your torso and legs in a straight line. This maintains core stability while moving the body around the elbow joint to target the biceps muscles.

This exercise can be adjusted to accommodate various levels of strength by using a taller table or chair to make the exercise easier, or a shorter table or chair to make the exercise more challenging. Depending on the type of chair or table, you might not be able to use a full range of motion if your head comes into contact with the bottom of the furniture. In this case, simply perform an isohold by holding the top position for a certain amount of time or perform a shorter-range pumping motion. Alternatively, grip both ends of a towel wedged into the top of a door. Use a neutral grip, which works the brachialis and brachioradialis a bit more than the biceps.

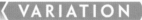 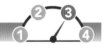

⟨ **VARIATION** ⟩

Long-Lever Inverted Curl

People who find this movement to be easy may lengthen the lever by performing the movement with straight legs that are elevated on to another chair or bench, thereby increasing the total percentage of body weight being lifted.

ARMS

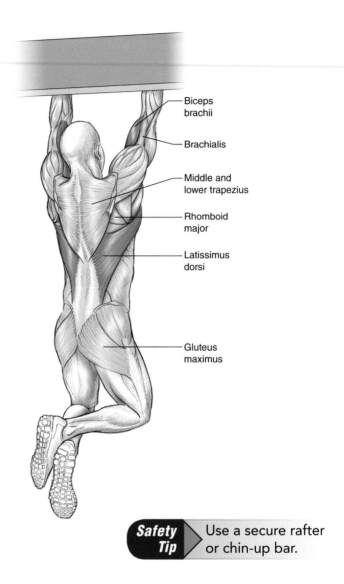

Biceps brachii

Brachialis

Middle and lower trapezius

Rhomboid major

Latissimus dorsi

Gluteus maximus

Safety Tip Use a secure rafter or chin-up bar.

Execution

1. Begin in a full-stretch position, hanging from a secure rafter or a chin-up bar with straight arms and a supinated grip, palms facing you. The toes will be off the ground and the knees can be bent if that's more comfortable.

2. Pull the body over the rafter or chin-up bar to sternum height while keeping the core stable.

3. Lower the body under control making sure you come all the way down.

Muscles Involved

Primary: Biceps brachii, latissimus dorsi

Secondary: Brachialis, lower and middle trapezius, rhomboids, rectus abdominis, gluteus maximus

Exercise Notes

The chin-up is a classic bodyweight exercise for the biceps and back muscles. A supinated grip with the palms facing you works the biceps the best, which is why this variation is included in the arms chapter. This movement requires a rafter or bar you can hang from with a supinated grip.

Many people perform this movement incorrectly by failing to use a full range of motion at the top and bottom of the movement, kicking their legs and using momentum, overarching their low back, and shrugging their shoulders at the top of the movement. Keep your core stable and your body in a straight line from the shoulders to the knees with a strong core and glute contraction. When at the very top of the movement with the chin over the bar, imagine tucking the shoulder blades into the back pockets so you keep them back and down. Use a full range of motion by starting from a dead stop position and rising all the way to where the rafter touches the top of your chest. If you perform chin-ups in this manner, you'll receive a very effective core workout in addition to a challenging upper-body workout.

ARMS

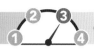

NARROW TRICEPS PUSH-UP

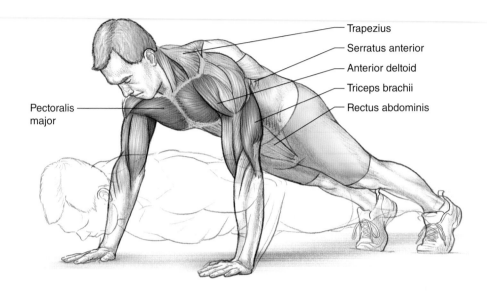

- Trapezius
- Serratus anterior
- Anterior deltoid
- Triceps brachii
- Rectus abdominis

Pectoralis major

Execution

1. Lie face down with the hands positioned shoulder-width apart and the elbows tucked into the body.

2. With the feet together and the core stable, press the body up.

3. Lower the body until the chest touches the floor.

Muscles Involved

Primary: Triceps brachii, pectoralis major, anterior deltoid

Secondary: Upper and lower trapezius, serratus anterior, rectus abdominis, gluteus maximus

Exercise Notes

The push-up performed with a narrow base is a classic exercise that targets the triceps and pectorals. No doubt it's extremely effective; however, most people perform this movement incorrectly by sagging at the hips, looking up and over-extending the neck, stopping short and failing to use a full range of motion, or failing to center their elbows over the wrists. Keep a strong core by flexing the abdominals and glutes. Keep the body in a straight line throughout the exercise and do not allow the hips to sag. Lower your body until the chest hits the floor.

Look down during the set and make sure the elbows are in line with the wrists. Keeping your body locked into a powerful position ensures that you receive a good core workout in addition to an effective upper-body workout.

Diamond Triceps Push-Up

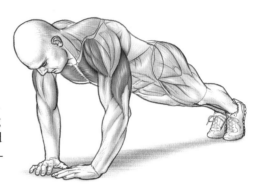

The diamond triceps push-up is a bit more challenging than the narrow triceps push-up because it relies more heavily on the triceps. This variation is performed with the hands touching each other and forming a diamond shape with the thumbs and index fingers.

 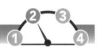
Short-Lever Triceps Push-Up

People who struggle with regular narrow triceps push-ups may shorten the lever by performing the movement from the knees. This reduces the total percentage of body weight being hoisted and allows for stricter form to be used.

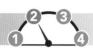
ARMS

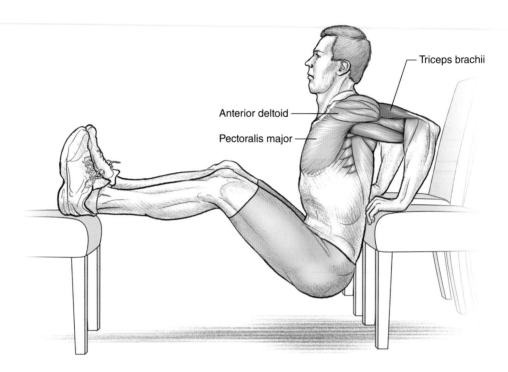

Triceps brachii

Anterior deltoid

Pectoralis major

Safety Tip Use sturdy, stable chairs or weight benches.

Execution

1. Set up three chairs so that your feet are resting on one and your body is centered between the other two. (If you have access to weight benches, you can perform this exercise using two weight benches. Set the benches parallel to each other. Place your palms on one bench and your heels on the other so your body is perpendicular to the benches.)

2. With your palms on the end of the two chairs, fingers forward, and your torso upright and legs in a straight line, lower the body under control until you receive an adequate stretch. Don't go too low; this could be dangerous. Upper arms parallel to the floor is deep enough.

3. Push your body up back to starting position.

Muscles Involved

Primary: Triceps brachii

Secondary: Pectoralis major, anterior deltoid

Exercise Notes

The bench dip is a common movement performed at gyms across the world. It's an effective triceps builder and can easily be adjusted depending on your strength level. Make the exercise easier by performing the movement with the feet flat on the floor and knees bent, which reduces the total amount of body weight being lifted. Descend deep enough to receive a good stretch in the muscles, but don't go too deep and place your soft tissue at risk. If you regularly descend too deeply, you risk injuring certain structures surrounding the shoulder joint. This exercise can be dangerous if not performed properly. Keep a tall chest during this movement and don't allow the lower back to round. Make sure you rise all the way to lockout.

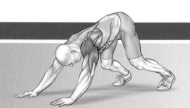

chapter 3

NECK AND SHOULDERS

Envision a strong, powerful man and he'll undoubtedly have a set of muscular shoulders and a thick neck. You'll never see a strong guy with wimpy shoulders or a puny neck. Moreover, thick shoulders create the illusion of a smaller waist, producing the coveted V taper. Although the latissimus dorsi (lats) are critical in creating this X factor, the top of the X actually starts with the deltoids (delts). The X factor is the coveted look men try to achieve. In order to achieve the X factor, a man needs strong upper-body musculature, a narrow midsection, and strong and muscular hips and thighs. The V taper, from the deltoids to the narrow midsection, characterizes a fit and athletic man.

Women often seek the defined and toned delts that signify a strong upper body, one built through hard work and effort. For many people, the shoulders can be stubbornly unresponsive to training, thereby requiring much devotion. To properly address the spectrum of shoulder and neck training, it's important that you understand the many functions of these muscles.

NECK

The neck is important in many sports. Collision sports such as American football, boxing, and rugby require strong necks to absorb strikes and prevent concussions or neck injuries. Grappling sports such as wrestling and Brazilian jiu-jitsu also require strong necks in order to prevent submissions and neck injuries.

Although the neck can move through all sorts of actions such as flexion, extension, lateral flexion, rotation, protraction, and retraction, we will focus primarily on strengthening the neck musculature isometrically during its forward (flexion) and backward (extension) motions. This will lead to a strong and stable neck, which is an overlooked aspect of spinal stability. Because these motions strengthen the various fibers of the trapezius and sternocleidomastoid, the scalenes, and the levator scapulae, the muscles responsible for other neck motions such as rotation and lateral flexion, you will cover all bases by performing these two movements.

Many assume that the only way to work the upper trapezius (figure 3.1) is through shrugging exercises that require scapular elevation. This is incorrect. The upper traps are heavily involved in upward rotation of the scapula and therefore get hit hard during handstand push-up motions. The same goes for the lower traps. In fact, you can adequately develop the fibers of the trapezius muscles by performing a balance of the horizontal and vertical pressing and pulling motions included in this book.

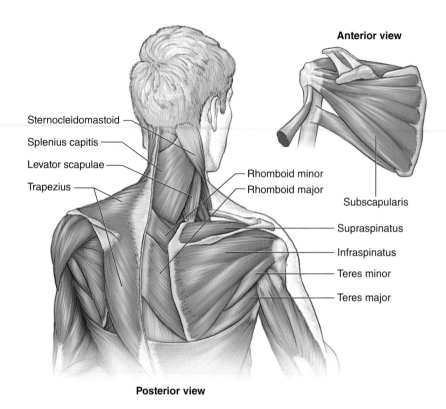

Anterior view

Sternocleidomastoid

Splenius capitis

Levator scapulae

Trapezius

Rhomboid minor

Rhomboid major

Subscapularis

Supraspinatus

Infraspinatus

Teres minor

Teres major

Posterior view

Figure 3.1   Neck and upper-back muscles.

Overhead pressing is complex in terms of biomechanics. Proper overhead pressing motions require adequate strength and mobility of the shoulder, upper back, and upper arm. When people work at a desk and sit for much of the day slumped over computers, posture erodes, which compromises lifting mechanics. For this reason beginners should stretch the upper body and progress gradually through the exercises to ensure that shoulder mobility and stability are developed in tandem. In particular, the upper spine should be able to extend and rotate properly and the shoulders should possess adequate mobility in all directions. Balanced strength and flexibility across the upper-body joints will keep the shoulders healthy and functioning properly throughout a lifetime.

SHOULDERS

The deltoids (figure 3.2) are important stabilizers of the glenohumeral joint and need to be strong and coordinated for rapid movement and for the prevention of shoulder dislocations. The deltoids contain three heads, each having a different function. When you get lean enough, you'll be able to see the three heads contracting while you train.

A well-developed middle head, or lateral deltoid, is the subdivision of the delts that leads to the illusion of the wide X shape mentioned earlier. The anterior head is on the front of the body, and posterior head is located on the back of

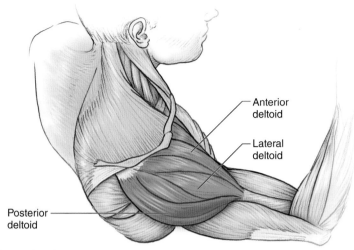

Figure 3.2 Deltoids.

the body. The anterior head is worked during push-up variations because it is a strong shoulder flexor and transverse, or horizontal, adductor. (Adduction moves a limb toward the midline of the body, and abduction moves a limb away from the midline of the body.) The posterior head is worked during various rowing and pull-up exercises because it acts as a shoulder extensor and transverse, or horizontal, abductor. However, this head is often underdeveloped. Specific attention to the rear delts is usually provided through transverse abduction movements of the shoulder. While all three heads contribute to handstand push-up movements, the anterior and lateral heads are worked the most during this category of lifts. The posterior head keeps the shoulder stable and contributes slightly to the overall motion.

Even if you were never to target your deltoids, you could achieve pretty good development by performing horizontal pressing and pulling movements such as push-ups and inverted rows. But to take your delt development to the next level, it is imperative to work them directly. There seemed to be fewer shoulder injuries many years ago when overhead pressing was more popular than horizontal pressing. This practice led to more stable shoulder muscles and balanced strength levels.

It should come as no surprise that the deltoids are heavily involved in sporting movements. They're involved in throwing jabs and crosses in boxing, chest passes in basketball, and pushing an opponent forward or stiff-arming an opponent in American football. In fact, the shoulders are heavily involved in all throwing, swinging, and striking motions predominant in sports such as baseball, tennis, racquetball, swimming, volleyball, and martial arts. The posterior deltoid is highly involved in the backhand stroke in tennis, a spinning backfist strike in mixed martial arts, rowing, or even a Frisbee serve. When carrying heavy loads at the sides of the body, the deltoids contract forcefully to keep the loads away from the body and prevent the humerus, the upper-arm bone, from pulling out of its socket.

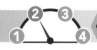
NECK

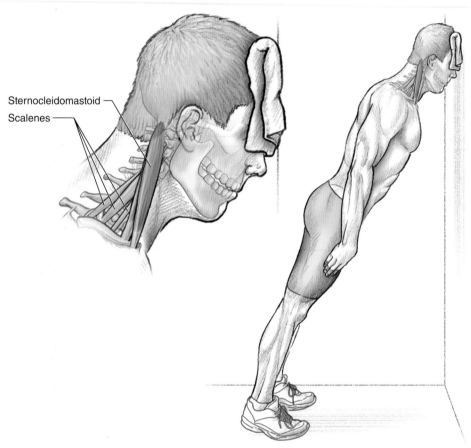

Sternocleidomastoid
Scalenes

Execution

1. Place a folded towel on the forehead.
2. From a standing position with arms at the sides, lean against the wall, making sure to keep the body in a straight line.
3. Hold for the desired amount of time.

Muscles Involved

Primary: Sternocleidomastoid
Secondary: Scalenes

Exercise Notes

The wall anterior neck isohold is an important exercise for proper neck muscle development. In collision and combat sports these muscles need to be strong because they're responsible for preventing neck hyperextension, which can occur during collisions or strikes if the muscles aren't sufficiently developed.

The difficulty of this exercise can be adjusted by moving up or down the wall. The farther up on the wall and the closer you stand to the wall, the easier it is, and the farther down on the wall and farther away you stand from the wall, the more challenging the exercise. I prefer to perform a 30-second hold, but you can opt for shorter or longer times depending on your goals.

Use a thick folded towel to cushion your head when you perform this movement. Keep your body in a straight line with a strong core and glute contraction.

⟨ **VARIATION** ⟩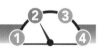

Wall Posterior Neck Isohold

The posterior neck isohold shifts the responsibility from the anterior neck musculature to the posterior neck musculature. This movement, which involves a neck extension hold, is carried out by the trapezius and cervical extensors. Perform this exercise for balanced neck strength.

Trapezius

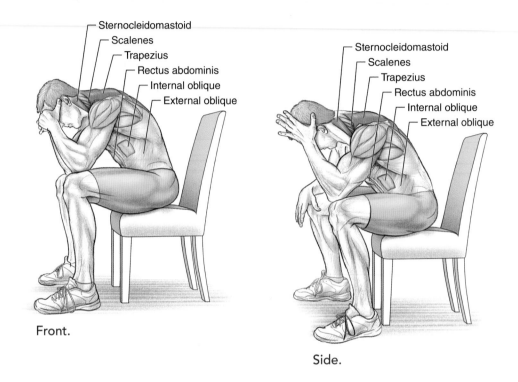

Front.

Side.

Execution

1. From a seated position with the elbows braced on the thighs, place the hands on the front of the head and apply manual (self-produced) isometric resistance for 10 seconds.

2. Place the hands on the back of the head and hold for another 10 seconds while applying manual resistance. If your arms are relatively short you may find that you have trouble keeping the elbows on the thighs for this variation.

3. Finish with a lateral isohold on each side (right and left) by placing the hand on the side of the head and applying manual resistance for 10 seconds.

Muscles Involved

Primary: Sternocleidomastoid, scalenes, trapezius, cervical extensors such as the semispinalis capitis and splenius capitis

Secondary: Rectus abdominis, internal and external obliques, erector spinae (spinalis, longissimus, iliocostalis)

Exercise Notes

Manual neck exercises are excellent for strengthening the neck musculature. Studies show that in order to strengthen the neck you have to train it directly. The neck muscles will not reach their maximum potential unless you perform specific neck exercises, and the good news is that it's very easy to train the neck through isometric holds.

Keep the neck in neutral position while you perform the holds. In neutral position, the neck is in its normal position, not twisted or tilted forward, backward, or to the side. Perform four holds: one for flexion, one for extension, one for right lateral flexion, and one for left lateral flexion.

A strong neck is important because it more securely connects the head to the torso, which reduces the risk of concussions.

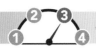
SHOULDERS

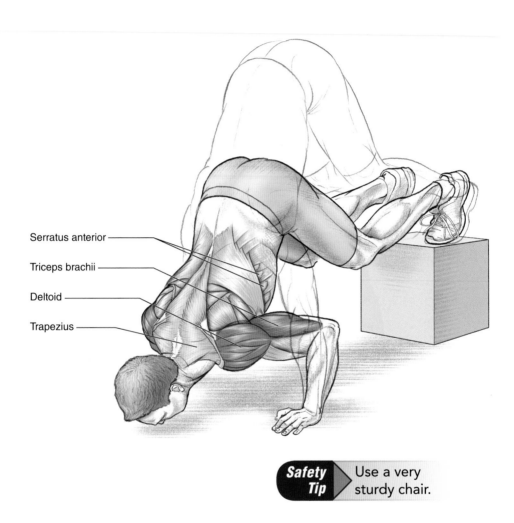

Serratus anterior

Triceps brachii

Deltoid

Trapezius

Safety Tip Use a very sturdy chair.

Execution

1. Place your hands on the floor just wider than shoulder width and your feet on top of a sturdy chair, box, or weight bench.

2. Pike up into an L-position by walking your hands back while flexing the hips and raising your buttocks toward the ceiling, then lower your body toward the floor by bending your elbows.

3. When your head reaches the ground, reverse the motion to starting pike position by locking out the arms and pushing the body high and away from the floor.

Muscles Involved

Primary: Deltoids, triceps brachii

Secondary: Upper and lower trapezius, serratus anterior

Exercise Notes

The feet-elevated pike push-up is an effective shoulder builder. Many people aren't quite strong enough to perform handstand push-ups, and the pike push-up is an excellent intermediate exercise in the progression to more challenging variations.

There is no need to hyperextend the neck in order to descend lower because the pike push-up is a partial-range movement no matter how you slice it. Keep your head and neck in neutral position and lower the body until the head touches the floor. Keep the body in an L-position throughout the movement.

⟨ VARIATION ⟩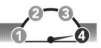

Three-Point Pike Push-Up

Once you become proficient in the feet-elevated pike push-up, increase the range of motion by performing the exercise between two sturdy, immobile chairs or boxes. This allows the head to travel farther down, placing more stress on the shoulder muscles and creating a more effective movement. The rear chair should be taller than the two front chairs.

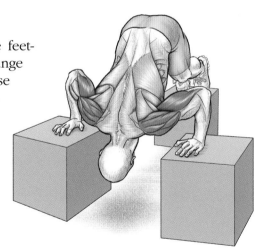

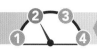
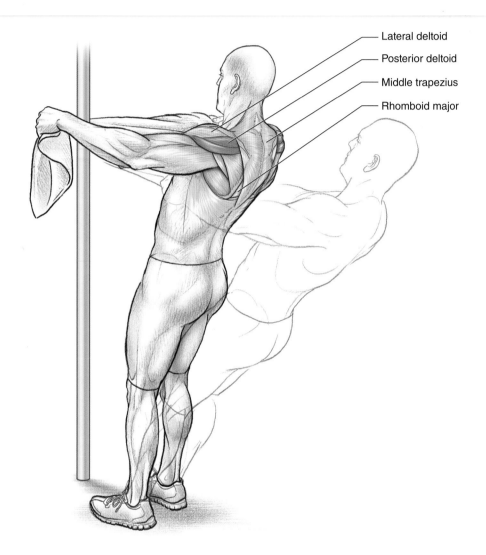

Lateral deltoid

Posterior deltoid

Middle trapezius

Rhomboid major

Execution

1. From a standing position with a towel wrapped around a pole, grab the ends of the towel and lean back into position.

2. Keeping the body in a straight line, raise your body by bringing the arms out to the sides.

3. Control the descent back to starting position.

Muscles Involved

Primary: Posterior deltoid

Secondary: Lateral deltoid, middle trapezius, rhomboid major

Exercise Notes

This move is easiest when you have a large towel and access to a pole. However, you have other options. You may also drape the end of a large towel over the top of a sturdy door and then shut the door, thereby wedging the towel into place. If the towel is wide enough, one will suffice, but two towels can be used as well. Keep your body in a straight line and focus on pulling the body up with the posterior deltoids and scapular retractors (middle trapezius and rhomboids). Adjust the level of difficulty by varying your body position. Stay more upright to make the exercise easier, and walk forward to create a greater trunk lean and more challenge.

Although this exercise has a short range of motion, it is important for balancing the shoulder musculature. Try your best to maintain tension on the posterior delts because these are often neglected and underdeveloped.

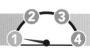
SHOULDERS

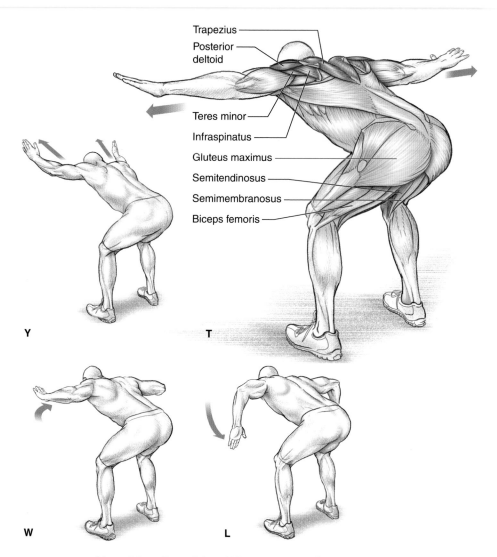

Trapezius

Posterior deltoid

Teres minor

Infraspinatus

Gluteus maximus

Semitendinosus

Semimembranosus

Biceps femoris

Y

T

W

L

Y position, T position, W position, and L position.

Execution

1. From a standing position, bend at the hips past a 45-degree torso angle, maintaining a neutral spine while sitting back and stretching the hamstrings.

2. Perform 10 dynamic Y motions by forming a Y with the arms, returning to starting position after each repetition. Switch to 10 T motions with the arms, followed by 10 W motions.

3. Transition into 10 L motions by holding the arms straight out with the elbows bent at 90 degrees and rotating at the shoulder joint so that the forearms move from vertical to the ground to parallel to the ground.

Muscles Involved

Primary: Lower trapezius, middle trapezius, rotator cuff musculature (infraspinatus, teres minor), posterior deltoid

Secondary: Hamstrings (biceps femoris, semitendinosus, semimembranosus), gluteus maximus

Exercise Notes

The YTWL is a terrific movement because it strengthens many of the crucial smaller muscles of the shoulder joint that provide stability and support for multi-joint movements. These muscles are not called on much during everyday activity so by activating them during the YTWL exercise, you'll prevent future injury or dysfunction. It is important to keep these muscles healthy.

You'll be surprised how challenging bodyweight resistance is throughout the set. Maintain good posture and don't allow the back to round.

SHOULDERS

Execution

1. Starting on your hands and knees, place your feet against the wall and walk your way up into a handstand position so that your toes end up against the wall, your body is relatively vertical and in a straight line, and you are facing the wall.

2. Lower the body slowly by bending the elbows until the head reaches the ground.

3. Reverse the movement and raise the body back to starting position. When the set finishes, walk your way down the wall back to your hands and knees.

Muscles Involved

Primary: Deltoids, triceps brachii

Secondary: Upper and lower trapezius, serratus anterior

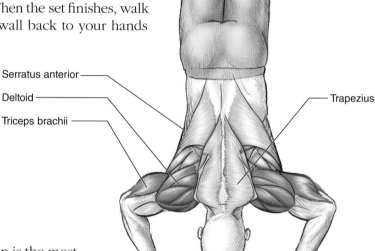

Serratus anterior

Deltoid

Triceps brachii

Trapezius

Exercise Notes

The wall handstand push-up is the most challenging overhead pressing movement because it requires you to lift your entire body weight. This exercise is much more challenging than a typical push-up for two reasons. First, people are stronger in horizontal pressing motions in comparison to vertical pressing motions. Second, the handstand push-up involves hoisting the entire body weight, whereas push-ups involve only about 70 percent because of the four points of contact with the floor and the angle of the torso.

There are several ways to perform this movement—feet against a wall behind the body, feet against a wall in front of the body, a partner holding the legs, or freestanding. Obviously the freestanding version is the most difficult because of balance requirements.

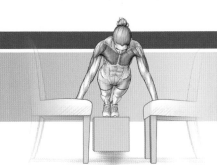

chapter 4

CHEST

There's a reason Mondays have been coined International Bench Press Day. Lifters around the world who desire well-developed pectorals prioritize their workouts by training their chests first each week. While most male exercisers are consumed with building the upper, middle, and lower areas of the pecs to their potential, women tend to be less concerned with chest development. However, a subtle line of muscle traversing the sternum can be quite attractive on a woman, and given that multijoint chest exercises also can serve as great triceps builders, it makes sense for women to incorporate pectoral movements into their routines.

Bodyweight training is well suited for chest training; all you need is a floor and you're good to go. It's essential that you pay attention to feeling the pectoral muscles working during multijoint pressing movements. Otherwise, the triceps and front deltoids can take over and rob the pecs of their neural activity. Bodybuilders refer to this as developing a mind–muscle connection, and it's one of the most important techniques you can use to enhance muscle development.

CHEST MUSCLES

The pectoralis major (figure 4.1) has three functional subdivisions—the upper, middle, and lower regions. The upper region is referred to as the sternoclavicular head because of its attachment to the clavicle, while the lower two regions are sometimes referred to as the sternocostal head because of their attachment at the ribs. To be even more accurate, researchers have found that the pectorals consist of six functional subdivisions that are recruited uniquely according to their lines of pull. The pectoralis major serves as a transverse adductor of the shoulder (used when throwing a ball sidearm), a shoulder adductor (used during a cable crossover), and internal rotator of the shoulder (used in arm wrestling).

The pectoralis minor is a small muscle under the pectoralis major that protracts, downwardly rotates, and depresses the scapula. It is trained during its stabilizing function during exercises such as dips. The pectoralis minor is often tight, which can alter posture and restrict proper scapular function during overhead pressing movements. For this reason it's a good idea to regularly perform pec stretches.

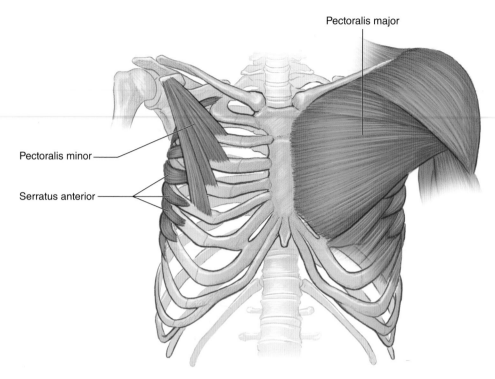

Figure 4.1   Muscles of the chest.

CHEST EXERCISES

For maximal pectoral development, a variety of chest exercises are warranted because certain exercises are better suited to developing the upper, middle, or lower regions. It may be possible to develop the inner and outer pectoral regions as well; however, research has failed to confirm this. Women who seek defined pecs should focus on upper-pectoral development because this area is more visible on a woman's body than the middle or lower pecs. Many men develop adequate middle and lower pectorals through frequent bench pressing and push-up performance and should focus on upper pectoral development for balanced aesthetics.

While the push-up, referred to as a press-up in some countries, is arguably the most popular bodyweight exercise and certainly the most common bodyweight chest exercise, it's important to progress to more challenging variations of the exercise for continued results. There are dozens of types of push-ups, and I have included the most effective push-up variations to allow you to achieve your goals.

Moreover, it's critical that you learn the proper way to perform a push-up from the get-go because a vast majority of exercisers perform this movement incorrectly. I distinctly remember when I started performing push-ups. I was 15 years old and could barely manage three sets of six repetitions. I'm pretty sure my form wasn't up to par back then either. Fortunately, I stuck with it and didn't

HALF PRICE BOOKS ®

Half Price Books
1835 Forms Drive
Carrollton, TX 75006
OFS OrderID   21624302

‖‖‖‖‖‖‖‖‖‖‖‖‖‖‖

SKU	ISBN/UPC	Title & Author/Artist	Shelf ID	Qty	OrderSKU
S34595019	9781450429290	Bodyweight Strength Training Anatomy Contreras, Bret	HLTH 3.1	1	

Thank you for your order, Valentina Lert!

Thank you for shopping with Half Price Books! Please contact service54@hpb.com. if you have
any questions, comments or concerns about your order (111-9870382-2337050)

SHIPPED STANDARD TO:
Valentina Lert
63357 RIDGE OVERLOOK CT
MONTROSE CO 81403-8471
vhnz51m89przybl@marketplace.amazon.com

ORDER# **111-9870382-2337050**
AmazonMarketplaceUS

‖‖‖‖‖‖‖‖‖‖‖‖‖

give up. Fast forward to today, I'm now able to perform 60 nonstop push-ups. A nice fringe benefit of push-up performance is the core stability that comes along with it.

The pectorals also are involved in many sport actions. Pushing opponents forward as in American football or sumo wrestling relies heavily on the pecs. Straight punching as in a jab or right cross involves the pecs, as does arced punching such as hooks or uppercuts. Tennis, volleyball, racquetball, and handball actions involving overhead and swinging motions across the body such as serving, forehand strokes, and spiking, involve the pectorals, as do throwing motions in baseball and American football. A shot-putter and discus thrower require strong and powerful pectorals to heave their implements the maximum distance. Mixed martial arts relies on the pecs for striking, clinching, takedowns, and grappling. Gymnasts and swimmers require strong pectorals for various maneuvers and strokes. Even track and field athletes train the pecs because a strong upper body can increase speed.

Some strength coaches prefer various types of push-up exercises to barbell bench pressing because they feel it's a safer and more natural movement pattern. Many feel that the requirements of the scapular stabilizers during the movement creates strong and healthy shoulders and safeguards against injury. The push-up is also a military training staple. Gymnasts are often able to perform a bench press with twice their body weight despite the fact that they never bench press; their extremely strong upper bodies are developed through frequent push-up and dip exercises and gruelling event practice. For optimal sport performance training, explosive pressing exercises are easy to perform through push-up movements that lend themselves to clapping and plyometric (repeated explosive movements) variations.

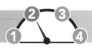
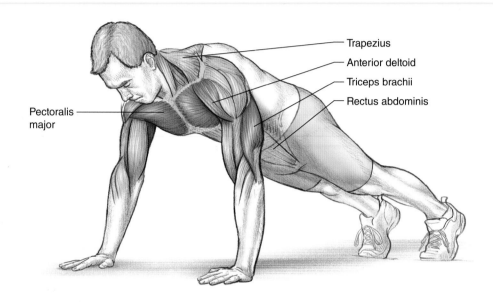

Trapezius

Anterior deltoid

Triceps brachii

Rectus abdominis

Pectoralis major

Execution

1. Place your hands slightly wider than shoulder width and your feet close together on the ground with your body in a straight line from heels to head.

2. With the arms at a 45-degree angle, the hands positioned directly under the elbows, the glutes and abs contracted, and the entire body tight, lower yourself until your chest touches the ground.

3. Reverse the movement and raise your body until your elbows lock out.

Muscles Involved

Primary: Pectoralis major, triceps brachii, anterior deltoid

Secondary: Serratus anterior, trapezius, rectus abdominis

Exercise Notes

Second to the biceps, the pectoralis major is the muscle men most want to develop, as evidenced by our obsession with push-ups and bench presses. But this exercise isn't all show and no go. Push-ups build upper-body strength and power, which transfers to punching and pushing power. Make this a full-body exercise by engaging the core and keeping the glutes squeezed as tightly as possible throughout the set. Many people sag at the hips, place their elbows too wide, and fail to use a full range of motion. By engaging the glutes and abs, you'll prevent the hips from sagging. Place your arms at a 45-degree angle from your body (abducted position) and make sure your forearms and hands are directly under the elbows for maximum shoulder joint health. Look down to keep the neck in neutral position. Lower all the way and come up all the way for correct performance, which allows you to also strengthen the shoulder stabilizers and keep the shoulders healthy for years to come.

⟨ VARIATION ⟩

Short-Lever Push-Up

The short-lever push-up is a good variation for beginners because it uses about 20 percent less body weight than a regular push-up, thereby making the exercise easier. Keep the arms tucked and the body straight as you perform the push-up from the knees.

⟨ VARIATION ⟩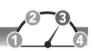

Wide-Width Push-Up

The wide-width push-up targets the pectoralis muscles differently than the regular push-up. To perform this movement, place the hands higher and wider on the floor compared to the standard version.

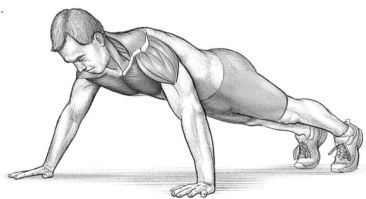

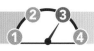

CHEST

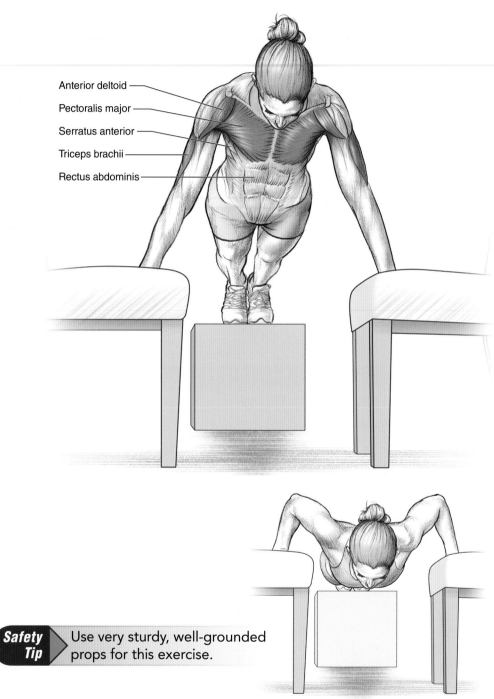

Anterior deltoid

Pectoralis major

Serratus anterior

Triceps brachii

Rectus abdominis

Safety Tip Use very sturdy, well-grounded props for this exercise.

Execution

1. Place your feet on top of a couch, chair, or box and your hands on top of two chairs positioned slightly wider than shoulder-width apart. You also could use objects such as a weight bench and two sturdy boxes.
2. Keeping the body in a straight line and glutes tight, descend until you feel a stretch in your pecs.
3. Reverse the movement and push your body up until your elbows lock out.

Muscles Involved

Primary: Pectoralis major, triceps brachii, anterior deltoid

Secondary: Serratus anterior, trapezius, rectus abdominis

Exercise Notes

The elevated push-up is an advanced variation of the push-up, allowing an increased range of motion at the shoulder joint. This equates to more muscle activation and ultimately more muscle mass. You don't want to aggravate the shoulder joint, so go only a few inches or centimeters deeper than you would during normal push-ups. The forearms should remain perpendicular to the floor and the hands placed at a medium width.

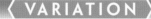 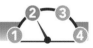

⟨ VARIATION ⟩

Short-Lever Elevated Push-Up

Exercisers who wish to take advantage of the extra range of motion provided in elevated push-ups but aren't quite strong enough to perform them can use the short-lever elevated push-up, which is performed with the knees, not the feet, on a couch or chair.

TORSO-ELEVATED PUSH-UP

CHEST

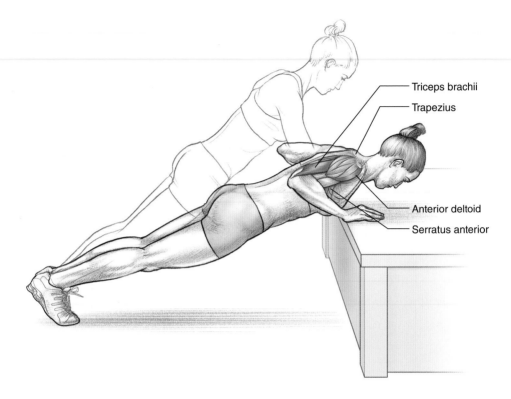

Triceps brachii

Trapezius

Anterior deltoid

Serratus anterior

Execution

1. Place your hands on top of a sturdy chair or table slightly wider than shoulder width and your feet close together on the ground.
2. Keeping your glutes contracted and your body in a straight line, lower yourself until your chest touches the chair or table.
3. Reverse the movement and raise your body until your elbows lock out.

Muscles Involved

Primary: Pectoralis major, triceps brachii, anterior deltoid

Secondary: Serratus anterior, trapezius, rectus abdominis

Exercise Notes

This is a great beginner variation because it allows you to perform the movement with proper core activation and accustoms you to keeping the body long and straight. As you progress, perform the movement from a lower table or chair to bring yourself closer to the ground. Eventually you'll be able to perform push-ups from the floor.

⟨ VARIATION ⟩

Feet-Elevated Push-Up

The feet-elevated push-up is an advanced pectoral exercise that uses a greater percentage of body weight and changes the angle to make the movement more like an incline press, thereby activating more upper-pectoral musculature. Although you need to go deep for maximal effectiveness, try not to look up too much at the bottom of the movement so you don't hyperextend the neck.

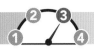
CHEST

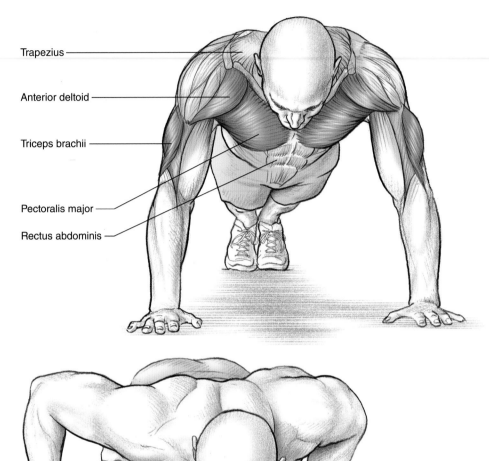

Trapezius

Anterior deltoid

Triceps brachii

Pectoralis major

Rectus abdominis

Descent to left side.

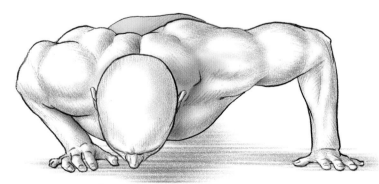

Descent to right side.

Execution

1. Begin in a standard push-up position, feet close together with toes on the floor, hands under shoulders.
2. As you descend into the push-up, lean to one side, placing more stress on the side that you're leaning toward.
3. Push up to lockout and alternate on the other side.

Muscles Involved

Primary: Pectoralis major, triceps brachii, anterior deltoid

Secondary: Serratus anterior, trapezius, rectus abdominis

Exercise Notes

The side-to-side push-up is an advanced variation that places more stress on the targeted side. The side you are targeting will take on about 65 percent of the load while the other side will take on about 35 percent. Moreover, this variation provides a challenging core workout because it's difficult to maintain proper body position throughout the movement. Try to resist excessive lateral and rotary spinal motion during the set.

⟨ VARIATION ⟩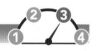

Sliding Side-to-Side Push-Up

You can use two paper plates on carpet to perform the sliding side-to-side push-up. (Also you could use commercially-available sliding exercise discs or, on a slick floor, small hand towels.) This is a highly challenging shoulder and core movement. Alternate hands, performing a push-up with one arm while sliding the other hand up in front of the body. Control the core and prevent excessive shifting and twisting.

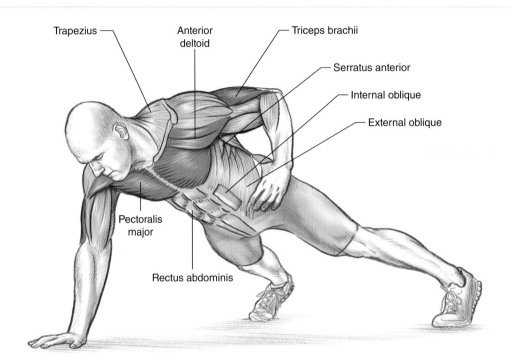

Trapezius

Anterior deltoid

Triceps brachii

Serratus anterior

Internal oblique

External oblique

Pectoralis major

Rectus abdominis

Execution

1. Take a wider-than-normal stance. Place one arm under your body and grab your upper outer leg with the nonworking arm.
2. Lower your body while keeping the grounded arm tucked in close to the torso, keeping the body straight, the core tight, and the hips square.
3. Lift yourself to lockout while preventing excessive lateral and twisting motions.

Muscles Involved

Primary: Pectoralis major, triceps brachii, anterior deltoid

Secondary: Serratus anterior, trapezius, rectus abdominis, internal oblique, external oblique

Exercise Notes

The one-arm push-up is the most challenging push-up variation included in this book. It is very difficult. Build up to performing this movement by starting with a short-lever position from the knees or from a torso-elevated position with the hand on a sturdy table or chair. Also you can simply lower your body by performing controlled negatives (lower yourself slowly) until you're able to push yourself back up properly. Control the side-to-side and rotary motions with strong core contractions.

⟨ **VARIATION** ⟩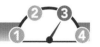

Self-Assisted One-Arm Push-Up

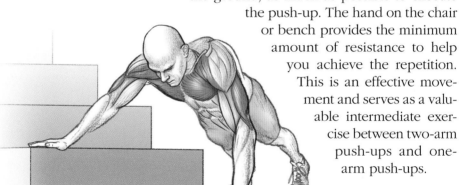

You can perform self-assisted one-arm push-ups by placing one hand on top of a sturdy chair, weight bench, or stair and relying on the other arm, hand on the ground, as much as possible to execute the push-up. The hand on the chair or bench provides the minimum amount of resistance to help you achieve the repetition. This is an effective movement and serves as a valuable intermediate exercise between two-arm push-ups and one-arm push-ups.

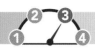
CLAPPING PUSH-UP

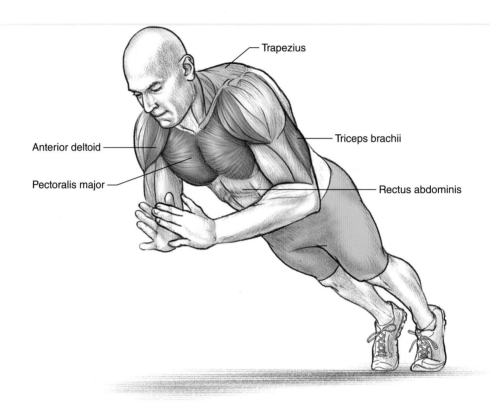

Trapezius

Triceps brachii

Anterior deltoid

Pectoralis major

Rectus abdominis

Execution

1. Begin in standard push-up position with feet close together and arms slightly wider than shoulder width.

2. Lower the body and then propel the body upward as forcefully as possible, keeping the feet on the ground.

3. Once airborne, clap the hands together and then catch the body in standard push-up position.

Muscles Involved

Primary: Pectoralis major, triceps brachii, anterior deltoid

Secondary: Serratus anterior, trapezius, rectus abdominis

Exercise Notes

The clapping push-up is an excellent upper-body plyometric movement that builds power and elastic strength in the shoulders, chest, and triceps. This is important for striking sports such as boxing and sports in which you push opponents forward such as American football. Do not let the quality of repetitions erode as the set progresses. Keep good form and make sure the movement stays athletic by sticking to fewer than six repetitions per set and focusing on maximum power generation.

〈 VARIATION 〉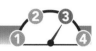

Knee Clapping Push-Up

People who struggle with clapping push-ups will find the knee clapping push-up easier. The variation shortens the lever and makes the movement easier since you perform this movement from the knees instead of the feet. But don't write this variation off as less effective than the standard clapping push-up. It uses less body weight, which means you can push your body up higher. Some folks are powerful enough to push their body back up to a tall kneeling position.

〈 VARIATION 〉

Whole-Body Clapping Push-Up

The whole-body clapping push-up is the most advanced variation of the mix because it requires incredible upper-body explosiveness and core strength. The goal is to spring the body upward with enough power to propel the entire body off the ground. Aim for maximum height and maintain the quality throughout the set. Land properly by having the feet touch the ground first and then absorbing the impact through eccentric contraction of the upper-body pressing muscles.

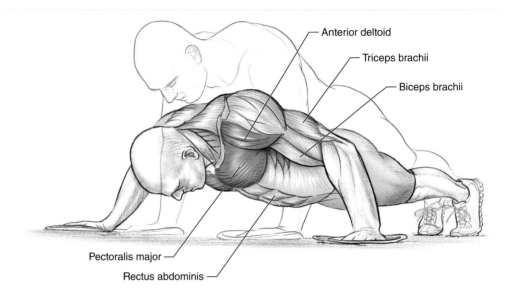

Anterior deltoid

Triceps brachii

Biceps brachii

Pectoralis major

Rectus abdominis

Execution

1. Begin in standard push-up position with both hands on paper plates, flared out slightly. Instead of paper plates, you also could use commercially-available sliding exercise discs or, on a slick floor, small hand towels.

2. Lower the body while sliding the arms out away from the body until the chest touches the floor.

3. Push the body up to starting position.

Muscles Involved

Primary: Pectoralis major, anterior deltoid

Secondary: Biceps brachii, triceps brachii, rectus abdominis

Exercise Notes

The sliding fly is an excellent way to target the pectorals. This movement is advanced and you may have to focus on controlled negatives, which involve lowering the body slowly, before you can perform them properly. In this case, you could perform a controlled negative from your feet and then drop to your knees and perform the concentric (positive) portion until you are able to do the exercise from the feet for the entire repetition. Make sure you're stretching the pecs and keeping the body in a straight line. Ensure that this movement is a fluid gliding motion and not choppy.

< VARIATION >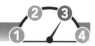

Short-Lever Sliding Fly

Another way to learn this movement is to shorten the lever and perform this movement from the knees instead of the feet. This will allow you to work your way up to performing standard repetitions and will allow you to use good form from the get-go.

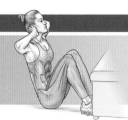

chapter 5

CORE

Core training has become an increasingly popular activity over the past decade, and for good reason. Sound core function is important for movement efficiency and joint health, not to mention injury prevention. And of course, there are the obvious effects on your appearance (after all, who doesn't covet six-pack abs?).

Putting together an optimal core training program requires three fundamental components: 1) an understanding of the muscles surrounding the core and the joint actions performed by the core, 2) knowledge of proper exercise form and volume prescription, and 3) the wisdom to tie it all together for maximal structural balance, muscular strength, and core stability. Accordingly, there has been a shift in the way fitness professionals have approached core programming over the years. We've gone from sit-ups to crunches to planks to now realizing that all types of core training can be beneficial, depending on the goals and abilities of the exerciser. The good news is that despite the fact that companies have made a killing through infomercials selling nifty abdominal exercise devices, research has consistently shown that all you need for a great core workout is your own body and a floor to lie on. Most infomercial products not only fail to outperform bodyweight movements in muscle activation, but they also are generally flimsy and awkward to use.

CORE MUSCLES

The definition of the core is a bit nebulous. Ask five personal trainers what comprises the core and you may get five different answers. Although most will agree that it includes the lumbar spine (low back), pelvis, and hip joints, there is little consensus on the specific musculature involved. Some say that it encompasses all the muscles between the knees and shoulders, while others feel that the core is limited to the muscles between the ribcage and pelvis. As you can see, determining the muscles of the core is a complicated process.

I classify the core into inner and outer muscles. The outer core includes the larger muscles such as the rectus abdominis, internal and external obliques, erector spinae, gluteus maximus, latissimus dorsi, quadratus lumborum, and psoas (figures 5.1 and 5.2). These muscles are primarily responsible for producing and resisting movement. The inner core muscles, on the other hand, form a cylinder that contracts just before and during limb movement to protect the spine by providing intra-abdominal pressure. These inner core muscles consist primarily of the multifidus in the rear, the transversus abdominis in the front and on the sides, the diaphragm up top, and the pelvic floor muscles on the bottom (figures 5.3 and 5.4).

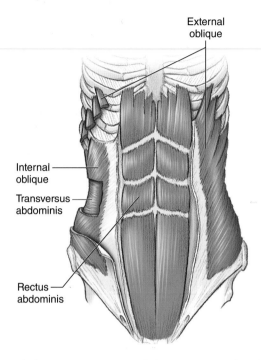

Figure 5.1   Rectus abdominis, transversus abdominis, internal and external obliques.

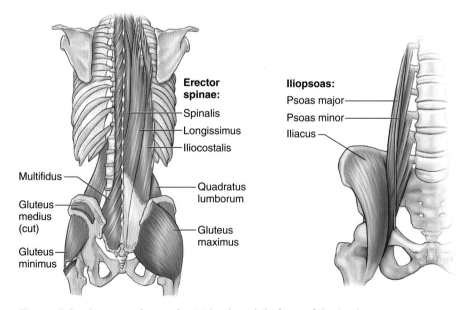

Figure 5.2   Core muscles on the (a) back and (b) front of the body.

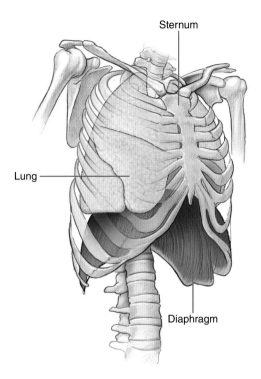

Figure 5.3 Diaphragm.

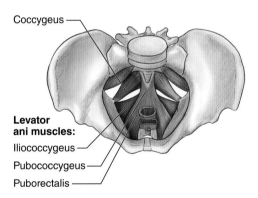

Figure 5.4 Pelvic floor muscles.

Dynamic core exercises—core exercises that involve movement such as spinal flexion, extension, lateral flexion, and rotation—are better suited for targeting individual muscles and teaching the core to produce and reduce force. Core stability exercises—core exercises that keep the spine in a static, or isometric, position—are better suited for teaching the body to resist movement and engage the inner core unit. Both types of exercises are important for optimal core function and performance.

CORE ACTIONS AND MOVEMENTS

The spine and pelvis work in combination to carry out movement. The lumbar spine can flex, extend, flex to either side, and rotate, while the pelvis can tilt to the front, back, and side and can rotate. And let's not forget the hips, which can flex, extend, abduct (move leg away from the middle), adduct (bring leg toward the middle), and internally and externally rotate. These actions require different muscle contributions to carry out the tasks. As you can imagine, many muscles are involved to varying degrees in the various joint actions of the core during activity.

In sports, the core is highly involved in nearly every movement. Force is transferred between the lower body and upper body through the core, so the core muscles must modulate their stiffness and timing in order to maximize the transfer of energy from one segment to the next. A weak core is not able to control excessive movement, which allows energy to leak instead of transferring it from one segment to the next.

The spine and pelvis move to various degrees during sporting movement. For example, during the stance phase of running when the body passes over the supporting foot, the lumbar spine typically extends while the pelvis tilts forward. During rotary actions such as swinging a bat, the front hip internally rotates while the back hip externally rotates, and the external oblique on one side and internal oblique on the other side contract to assist this rotation through a stiff core. Ample motion at the hips and thoracic spine (upper back) limit the amount of rotation in the low back while transferring energy from the hips to the upper extremities. The lumbar spine (low back) must be strong enough to resist being extended during collision sports such as football and rugby. The core is highly involved in all major sporting movements that happen when your feet are primarily on the ground, such as sprinting, jumping, twisting, throwing, and cutting from side to side. It is also involved in other sporting movements, such as swimming.

Strong core muscles play a role in posture, as well. In particular, the erectors must be strong to prevent thoracic kyphosis (hunchback), and the abdominals must be strong enough to prevent lumbar lordosis (swayback) and excessive anterior pelvic tilt. Maintaining a balanced core strength helps the body properly distribute forces during heavy and explosive movement, which spares the spine and prevents low back pain.

CORE EXERCISES

This chapter contains a variety of core exercises that will improve your ability to produce motion through concentric power, resist motion through isometric power, and absorb or decelerate motion through eccentric power. Each of these qualities is important in sports and functional movement. Not only does the chapter contain a balance of dynamic and static, or isometric, exercises, it also varies exercises in terms of planes and directions of movement. For example, frontal plane exercises are well suited for transferring to lateral movement, sagittal plane exercises are well suited for transferring to forward and backward movement, and transverse plane exercises are well suited for transferring to rotary movement. Finally, the chapter contains a balance of beginner and advanced exercises to accommodate a wide range of ability and to allow for the development of power, strength, and strength endurance in addition to well-developed abs.

You must understand correct exercise technique for the different areas of your core. Your hips and thoracic spine (upper back) should be mobile and move efficiently; however, you should limit spinal motion in the lumbar region. For example, when performing crunches and side crunches, your upper back should move the most while the lower back, or lumbar spine, moves the least. It is also essential to maintain good posture during core-stability exercises. Proper body position while you're building isometric strength and endurance will transfer to the field, so be aware of what your body looks like when holding core-stability exercises.

CORE

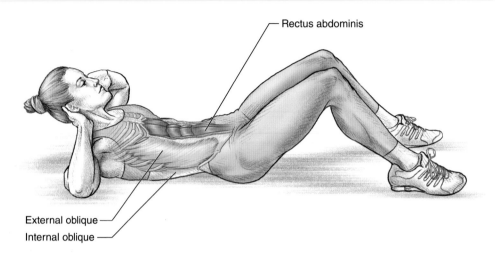

Rectus abdominis

External oblique

Internal oblique

Execution

1. Lie supine with the knees bent, feet on the floor, and hands at the ears. Hold the head and neck in neutral position, not flexed or twisted.

2. Flex the spine to 30 degrees of trunk flexion with most of the motion occurring in the thoracic spine, keeping the head and neck in proper position.

3. Hold at the top briefly and then lower the trunk slowly under control.

Muscles Involved

Primary: Rectus abdominis

Secondary: External oblique, internal oblique

Exercise Notes

The crunch is one of the most basic core exercises in the books. It targets the muscles of the abdominal wall and strengthens the dynamic trunk-flexion role of the core, which is critical for sport actions such as throwing a baseball, serving a tennis ball, or spiking a volleyball.

Limit the flexion of the low back during the crunch and focus most of the motion in the upper back. Raise the torso to just 30 degrees of total trunk flexion and make sure you accentuate the isometric portion (the static hold when you keep the body motionless) at the top as well as the eccentric (lowering) component.

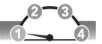
Reverse Crunch

While the standard crunch targets the upper rectus abdominis a bit better than the lower rectus abdominis, if done correctly the reverse crunch will recruit more lower rectus abdominis and oblique activity because of the posterior pelvic tilting involved in the variation. Start with the hips flexed at 90 degrees and knees bent. Pull the knees toward the head and raise the buttocks off the ground.

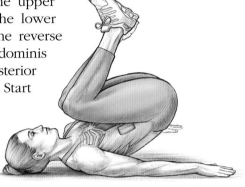

Side Crunch

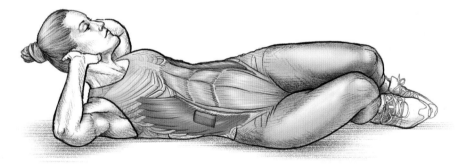

The side crunch variation is performed by shifting onto your side with the hips flexed and raising the trunk to about 30 degrees of lateral trunk flexion. Performing the crunch in this manner targets the obliques.

CORE

CORE

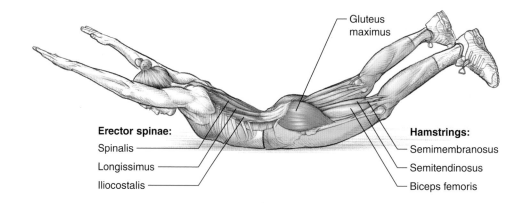

Gluteus maximus

Erector spinae:
Spinalis
Longissimus
Iliocostalis

Hamstrings:
Semimembranosus
Semitendinosus
Biceps femoris

Execution

1. Lie prone on the ground with the arms stretched forward in front of the body, palms down, and the knees slightly bent and shoulder-width apart.

2. Simultaneously raise the torso and legs off the ground, hyperextending at the hips and not just the spine. Target the glutes and hamstrings in addition to the spinal erectors.

3. Hold the top position briefly and then lower the body to starting position.

Muscles Involved

Primary: Gluteus maximus, erector spinae (spinalis, longissimus, iliocostalis)

Secondary: Hamstrings (biceps femoris, semitendinosus, semimembranosus)

Exercise Notes

The superman exercise is an awesome core exercise if performed properly. Many use poor form by overextending the lower back and trying to isolate the erector spinae. This is not ideal. The exercise is more productive if you limit the amount of lumbar hyperextension and instead attempt to hyperextend the hips by squeezing the gluteals and hamstrings and raising the legs off the ground. Elevate the legs and torso to about a 20-degree angle relative to the ground and rely heavily on the gluteals.

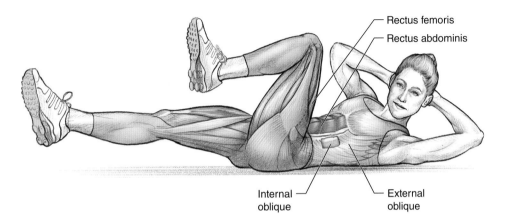

Rectus femoris

Rectus abdominis

Internal oblique

External oblique

Execution

1. Lie supine with the hips flexed in the air at 90 degrees.
2. With the hands at the ears, flex and rotate the upper spine by raising the torso off the ground about 30 degrees and twisting while flexing the opposite hip until the elbow and opposite knee meet each other.
3. Reverse the movement and twist to the opposite side as if riding a bicycle.

Muscles Involved

Primary: Rectus abdominis, psoas, rectus femoris

Secondary: Internal oblique, external oblique

Exercise Notes

The bicycle is an effective abdominal movement that works the core in several capacities, including trunk flexion, trunk rotation, and hip flexion. The motion requires a balance of strength and coordination. Once you get the hang of it you'll feel it working the entire core. Don't move too much at the lumbar spine. Rise up just enough to lift your shoulder blades off the floor.

CORE

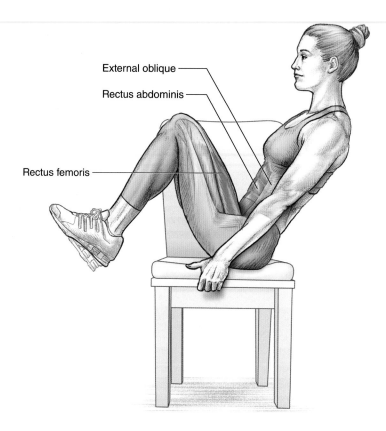

External oblique

Rectus abdominis

Rectus femoris

Execution

1. While seated, lean back and grab the seat of the chair, keeping the feet on the floor, chest up, and head and neck in neutral position.
2. Keeping the knees bent, simultaneously move the trunk forward and the legs upward so the trunk and thighs move toward each other.
3. Lower the torso and feet to starting position.

Muscles Involved

Primary: Rectus abdominis, psoas, rectus femoris

Secondary: Internal oblique, external oblique

Exercise Notes

Strong hip flexor muscles power the legs upward while running. While the rectus femoris is more active in lower ranges of hip flexion, as the hips rise the psoas become more important. The seated knee-up strengthens the abdominals and hip flexors together to help produce a strong anterior chain. Maintain good posture throughout this movement by keeping the chest tall and head and neck in neutral position.

〈 VARIATION 〉

L-Sit

The L-sit is a challenging variation that involves holding an isometric, 90-degree, hips-flexed position while the entire body hovers over the ground. This advanced variation can be attempted after you've gained sufficient core strength and hamstring flexibility through other exercises. If you have proportionally shorter arms, you can place two blocks next to you, and you can put your palms flat on the blocks.

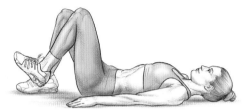

CORE

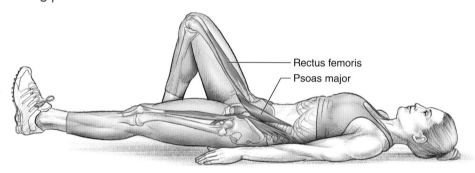

Starting position.

Rectus femoris
Psoas major

Execution

1. Lie supine (face-up) on the ground. Bend both knees. Plant one foot on the ground and lift the other in the air, keeping the hip and knee flexed at 90 degrees.

2. Lower the bent leg toward the ground. As it approaches the ground, straighten the knee as you continue lowering the leg toward the ground, stopping just short of contact. Keep your lumbar spine in neutral position.

3. Reverse the movement and return to starting position.

Muscles Involved

Primary: Lower rectus abdominis, psoas major, rectus femoris

Secondary: Upper rectus abdominis, internal oblique, external oblique

Exercise Notes

The bent-knee single-leg lowering with extension exercise is an excellent beginner exercise for increasing stability of the low back and pelvis by strengthening the hip flexors and abdominals. This exercise looks easy, but if you do it properly you'll realize that it isn't. Many people fail to maintain proper lower-back alignment throughout this exercise. It's critical that you learn to stabilize the spine properly during these types of movements.

⟨ VARIATION ⟩

Dead Bug

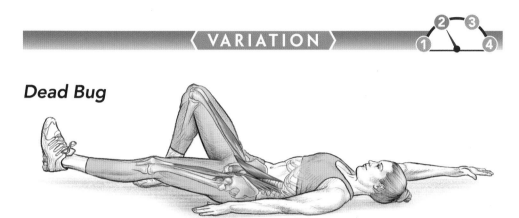

The dead bug exercise is a more challenging variation that involves diagonal arm and leg movements. Start in a supine position with the hips, knees, and shoulders flexed to 90 degrees. Simultaneously lower one leg and the opposite arm toward the floor while keeping the lower back in a neutral position. This is much harder than it appears.

DOUBLE-LEG LOWERING WITH BENT KNEES

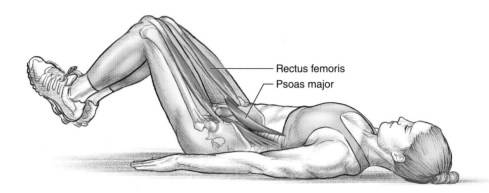

Rectus femoris
Psoas major

Execution

1. Lie supine, palms down and neck in neutral position, with hips and knees flexed to 90 degrees.
2. Keeping the knees bent, slowly lower both feet to the floor through eccentric hip extension. Do not let the lower back flatten out.
3. Reverse the movement to return to starting position.

Muscles Involved

Primary: Lower rectus abdominis, psoas major, rectus femoris

Secondary: Upper rectus abdominis, internal oblique, external oblique

Exercise Notes

The double-leg lowering with bent knees exercise is another challenging core-stability exercise that involves flexing and extending the hips while keeping the lumbar spine in neutral position. The low back will want to overarch and the pelvis will want to anteriorly rotate, but you will resist this motion and teach the spine to remain stable under strong extension torque. Perform this movement slowly and under control and you'll be able to feel the correct muscles working.

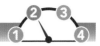

Lying Straight-Leg Raise

The lying straight-leg raise is an advanced variation of double-leg lowering movements. Most people perform the movement incorrectly. Keep good posture during this movement and lower the legs slowly and under control.

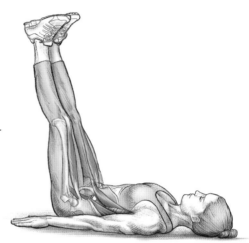

Dragon Flag

The dragon flag is a highly advanced variation. Make sure you're able to perform simpler movements before attempting this movement. Lie supine and grab hold of an object behind you such as a pole or bottom of a stable chair. Rotate your entire body about your upper shoulders, keeping the body in a straight line and maintaining good posture and core contraction.

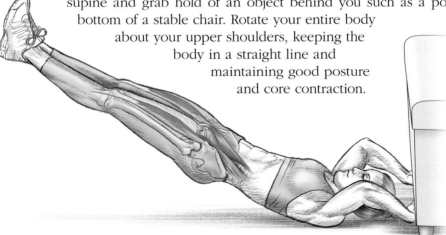

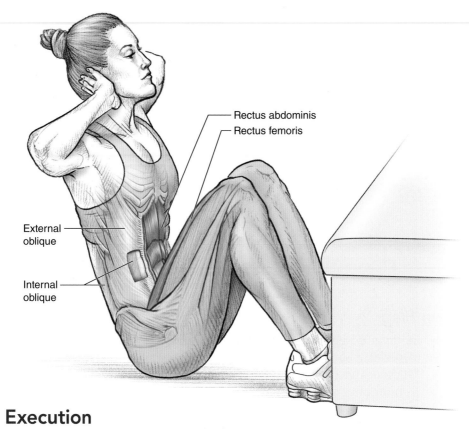

Rectus abdominis
Rectus femoris
External oblique
Internal oblique

Execution

1. Lie supine with the hips bent 45 degrees and knees bent 90 degrees.
2. With the hands at the ears, flex the hips and upper back while moving only slightly in the lumbar spine.
3. Return to starting position.

Muscles Involved

Primary: Rectus abdominis, psoas, rectus femoris

Secondary: Internal oblique, external oblique

Exercise Notes

The bent-knee sit-up is a classic core exercise but many people do more harm than good with this movement by flexing too much at the lumbar spine. Maintain proper lumbar posture throughout the movement by bending at the hips and upper back and limiting the range of motion in the low back. You can hook the feet under a sofa or something heavy to allow more torque production at the hips. Perform the movement under control and accentuate the negative portion (lowering component) of the exercise rather than cranking out 100 repetitions in a ballistic manner.

⟨ VARIATION ⟩

Straight-Leg Sit-Up

The straight-leg sit-up is a variation of the sit-up and requires hamstring flexibility. Use the hip flexors to pull your body up while keeping the chest tall to prevent excessive rounding of the lower back.

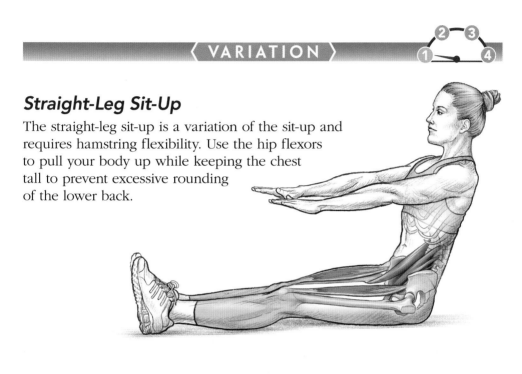

⟨ VARIATION ⟩

Twisting Sit-Up

The twisting sit-up is another classic movement, but just like the other sit-up variations, make sure you're performing the exercise correctly. As you rise, keep the chest up to prevent excessive rounding. Don't overrotate. Bring the opposite elbow toward the knee at the top of the movement.

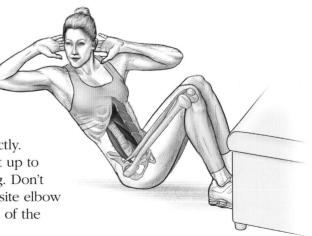

FRONT PLANK

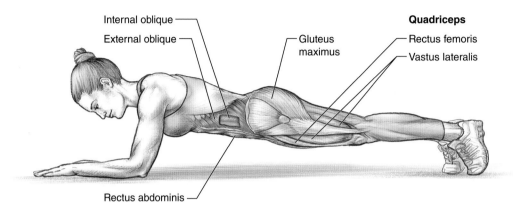

Internal oblique
External oblique
Gluteus maximus
Quadriceps
Rectus femoris
Vastus lateralis
Rectus abdominis

Execution

1. Form a pillar or bridge by supporting your body in a prone position with only the feet and forearms touching the ground.

2. Keeping the body in a straight line with the elbows directly beneath the shoulders, the hands flat on the floor or clasped, and the head looking down, forcefully contract the quads and glutes.

3. Hold for time. Depending on your fitness level, hold the position for 30 seconds to 3 minutes.

Muscles Involved

Primary: Rectus abdominis, internal oblique, external oblique

Secondary: Gluteus maximus, quadriceps (rectus femoris, vastus lateralis, vastus medialis, vastus intermedius)

Exercise Notes

The front plank is the most basic core-stability exercise. Unfortunately it is often performed improperly. Contract the quads to straighten the knees. Keep the body in a straight line. Many people either allow the hips to sag or bow up into an upside down V position. Look down to avoid hyperextending the neck. Finally, squeeze the glutes to posteriorly rotate the pelvis. This makes the movement much more challenging for the glutes, abdominals, and obliques. When performed in this manner, the movement is challenging. It's not uncommon to experience shaking and trembling after only 15 seconds.

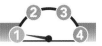
Short-Lever Front Plank

Beginners can practice proper plank performance by shortening the lever and conducting the exercise from their knees. The same rules apply. Make sure the body is in a straight line from the shoulders to the knees and squeeze the glutes.

⟨ VARIATION ⟩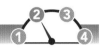

Feet-Elevated Front Plank

It is possible to make the static hold more challenging by elevating the feet onto a weight bench, sturdy chair, or small table. Just don't elevate the body too high. Ideally you want to be parallel to the ground for a maximum challenge.

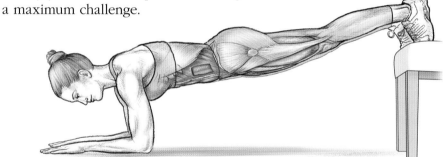

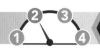

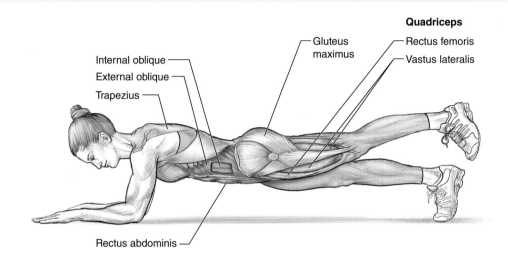

Quadriceps

Gluteus maximus — Rectus femoris — Vastus lateralis

Internal oblique — External oblique — Trapezius

Rectus abdominis —

Execution

1. Get into a standard plank position. While keeping the body stable, lift an arm into the air and hold for a 1-second count.
2. Return to starting position then raise the other arm into the air while keeping the body stable.
3. Return to starting position then raise one leg.
4. Return to starting position and raise the other leg.
5. Continue to rotate limbs in this manner for the entire set.

Muscles Involved

Primary: Rectus abdominis, internal oblique, external oblique

Secondary: Gluteus maximus, quadriceps (rectus femoris, vastus lateralis, vastus medialis, vastus intermedius), trapezius

Exercise Notes

It is important to continually challenge the body. The standard plank, while an excellent exercise for beginners, is too easy for intermediate and more advanced exercisers. One way to make the exercise more difficult is to raise one limb off the floor during the plank, thereby decreasing stability and introducing a rotary stability challenge to the spinal column. The key is to keep the body stable, preventing any leaning or twisting action in the trunk, while moving the limbs off the ground. Aim for a 60-second set.

⟨ VARIATION ⟩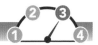

Rotating Two-Point Plank

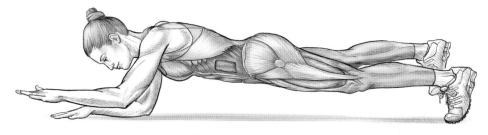

When the rotating three-point plank is mastered, it is possible to make the exercise even more challenging by performing a rotating two-point plank. Simply raise one arm and the opposite leg at the same time while keeping the body stable and preventing motion at the pelvis and spine.

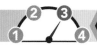
CORE

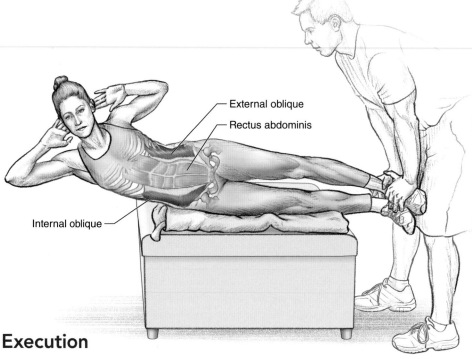

External oblique

Rectus abdominis

Internal oblique

Execution

1. Begin with a partner holding your feet, your lower body draped over a weight bench, small table, or loveseat in a side-lying position, and your upper body suspended in the air with the hands at the ears and legs straight.

2. Lower the torso toward the floor, limiting the bending in the lower spine while receiving a stretch in the upper hips. Avoid rotating during the movement.

3. Raise the torso with a strong contraction in the gluteus medius and obliques.

Muscles Involved

Primary: External oblique, internal oblique, gluteus medius, quadratus lumborum

Secondary: Rectus abdominis, erector spinae (spinalis, longissimus, iliocostalis), multifidus

Exercise Notes

The partner-assisted oblique raise is a challenging movement that requires a partner. Make sure the partner is well positioned and able to hold your lower body in position and keep your feet stationary. Make this a hips-and-core movement rather than just bending at the low back. The motion is completely lateral and medial; there should be no twisting or bending forward at the hips during the movement. Cross the arms in front of the body and when that becomes easy, place the hands overhead in a prisoner position (hands behind the head and elbows out) to make the movement more challenging.

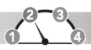

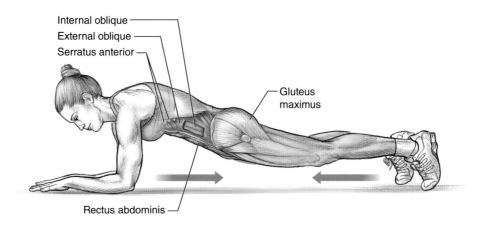

Internal oblique
External oblique
Serratus anterior
Gluteus maximus
Rectus abdominis

CORE

Execution

1. Get into standard plank position on the forearms and toes.
2. Squeeze the glutes as hard as possible to posteriorly tilt (tuck under) the pelvis. Hold the pelvic tuck throughout the duration of the set.
3. Try to drive the elbows to the feet and the feet to the elbows as if trying to pike upward but keep the body in good alignment.

Muscles Involved

Primary: Rectus abdominis, external oblique, internal oblique

Secondary: Gluteus maximus, serratus anterior

Exercise Notes

The RKC plank is an intermediate plank variation that requires considerable muscle skill and endurance. Many people lack the abdominal and gluteal motor skills and stamina to produce a pelvic tuck (posterior tilt) and hold it for time. It is important to be able to dissociate the pelvis from the spine and to possess strong glutes because they help prevent excessive anterior (forward) tilt or over-arching. This variation builds gluteal endurance as well as lower abdominal and oblique endurance. The key is to hold the pelvic tilt while driving the elbows toward the feet and the feet toward the elbows, making the isohold considerably more challenging. It takes time to master this movement, so make sure you're proficient in simpler plank variations before attempting the RKC plank.

SIDE PLANK

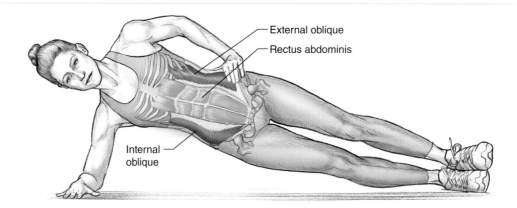

External oblique

Rectus abdominis

Internal oblique

Execution

1. Form a side pillar or bridge by supporting your body in a side-lying position with just one foot and one forearm touching the ground. Stack the legs and place the hand of the upper arm on the hip.
2. Keep the body in a straight line from head to foot with a neutral head and neck position. Squeeze the glutes and keep the forearm of the lower arm pointed straight ahead.
3. Hold for time. Depending on your exercise level, hold for 15 to 60 seconds.

Muscles Involved

Primary: External oblique, internal oblique, gluteus medius, quadratus lumborum

Secondary: Rectus abdominis, erector spinae (spinalis, longissimus, iliocostalis), multifidus

Exercise Notes

The side plank is an incredibly functional exercise that trains the obliques and gluteus medius in an isometric fashion, which is akin to their stabilizing role during many dynamic activities. Keep the entire body in neutral position and keep the core and glutes tight. Many people unknowingly lean forward or backward, set up in a twisted position, or bend at the hips when performing this movement. This is a core-stability exercise, so you need to resist motion and keep your body in a long, athletic position.

CORE

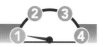
Short-Lever Side Plank

People who struggle with the conventional side plank should master the short-lever side plank before moving on to the side plank. Because the exercise is performed from the knees rather than from the feet, a lower percentage of body weight is used and the exercise is easier to control. The same rules apply: stay long and motionless.

 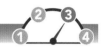
CORE

Feet-Elevated Side Plank

The feet-elevated side plank is an advanced variation of the side plank. Elevate the feet onto a weight bench, small chair, box, or sturdy table. Ideally, you want the body to be parallel to the floor. Make the exercise even more challenging by combining a hip abduction (like a side-lying hip raise) with the top leg or an external hip rotation (like a side-lying clams) while holding the position.

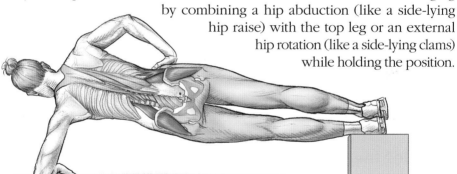

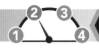

CORE

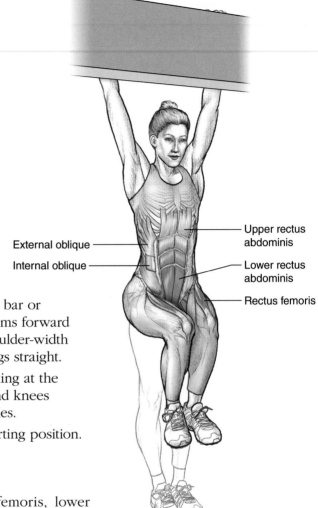

External oblique

Internal oblique

Upper rectus abdominis

Lower rectus abdominis

Rectus femoris

Execution

1. Hang from a chin-up bar or sturdy rafter with palms forward and hands about shoulder-width apart, keeping the legs straight.

2. Raise the legs by flexing at the hips until the hips and knees are at 90-degree angles.

3. Lower the legs to starting position.

Muscles Involved

Primary: Psoas, rectus femoris, lower rectus abdominis

Secondary: Upper rectus abdominis, internal oblique, external oblique, anterior and posterior forearm muscles (such as the flexor carpi radialis and palmaris longus), lower trapezius

Exercise Notes

The rafter-hanging leg raise with bent knees is a great hip flexor exercise that should help you reposition your legs faster when sprinting. Keep the lumbar spine in neutral position during this movement by moving mostly in the hips and upper back and not so much in the lower back. All the motion occurs at the hips. Lift the knees just until the upper thighs are parallel to the floor and then lower the legs.

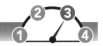

Straight-Leg Hanging Leg Raise

The straight-leg hanging leg raise is an advanced variation that requires excellent hip flexor strength and hamstring flexibility. The same rules apply: keep the lumbar spine stable while moving solely at the hips.

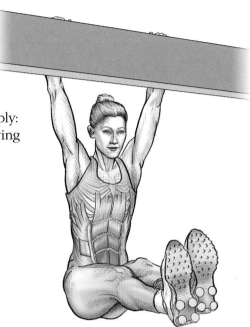

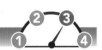

Hanging Leg Raise With Reverse Crunch

The hanging leg raise with reverse crunch combines hip flexion, posterior pelvic tilt, and lumbar flexion to work the hip flexors and abdominals. Raise the knees. When you reach 90 degrees, keep raising by titling the pelvis back and flexing the spine a bit, which will allow you to bring the knees all the way up toward your shoulders.

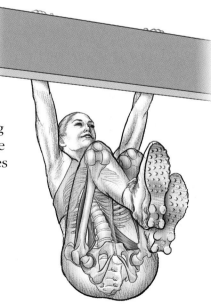

CORE

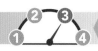
OBLIQUE HANGING LEG RAISE

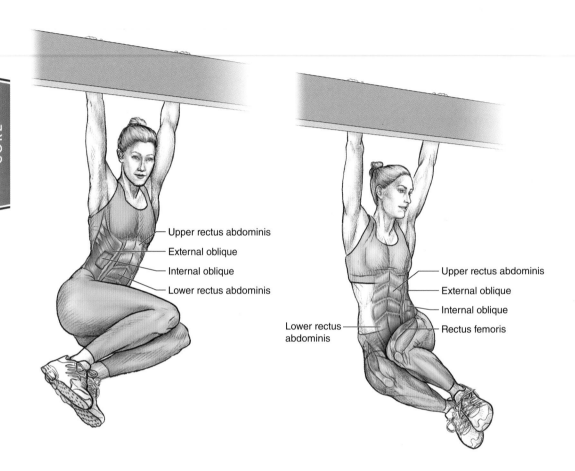

Upper rectus abdominis
External oblique
Internal oblique
Lower rectus abdominis

Upper rectus abdominis
External oblique
Internal oblique
Lower rectus abdominis
Rectus femoris

Execution

1. Hang from a chin-up bar or sturdy rafter with knees bent and hands shoulder-width apart, palms facing forward. Raise the knees by flexing at the hips. At the same time, pull your knees to one side by laterally flexing the spine.

2. Raise the knees to slightly over 90 degrees relative to the ground. Lower the legs to starting position then alternate to the other side.

Muscles Involved

Primary: Internal oblique, external oblique, psoas, rectus femoris, lower rectus abdominis

Secondary: Upper rectus abdominis, anterior and posterior forearm muscles (such as the flexor carpi radialis and palmaris longus), lower trapezius

Exercise Notes

The oblique hanging leg raise is a challenging core exercise that works the entire anterior core with special emphasis on the obliques. Make sure you're proficient in side crunches and other simpler oblique movements before attempting this exercise. Control the motion and ensure that it is smooth.

⟨ VARIATION ⟩

Windshield Wiper

The windshield wiper is an extremely advanced exercise. Don't try it until you have mastered more basic core movement patterns. To perform this movement, raise the legs toward the

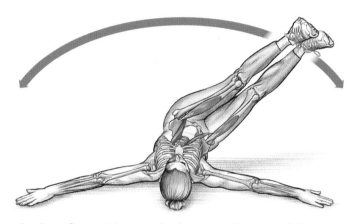

shoulders and then rotate the legs from side to side, keeping the core tight and twisting mostly with the upper back, not the lower back. Control the motion and limit the rotational range of motion to spare the spine.

CORE

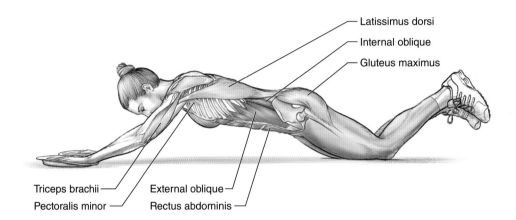

Latissimus dorsi

Internal oblique

Gluteus maximus

Triceps brachii

Pectoralis minor

External oblique

Rectus abdominis

Execution

1. Assume a kneeling position with both hands on paper plates. You may also use commercially-available sliding exercise discs or, on a slick floor, small hand towels. Squeeze the glutes and keep the head and neck in a neutral position.

2. Lower your body under control by extending the hips and flexing the arms until your body approaches the floor. Keep the glutes contracted forcefully.

3. Rise back to the starting position.

Muscles Involved

Primary: Rectus abdominis, internal oblique, external oblique

Secondary: Gluteus maximus, latissimus dorsi, triceps brachii, pectoralis minor

Exercise Notes

The rollout is one of the best core stability exercises. If you use proper form and keep the glutes contracted, preventing the pelvis from rotating forward, your lower abdominals will receive even more of a workout, and you are likely to be sore for quite a while if you aren't accustomed to the movement. Break into this exercise gradually and make sure you keep the body in a straight line at the bottom of the movement. Many people sag at the hips or allow too much anterior pelvic tilt during the rollout exercise.

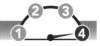
Standing Rollout

Once you've mastered the kneeling rollout, you can progress to the standing rollout, one of the most challenging core movements around. From a standing position, reach down and place your hands on paper plates or other sliding devices. Slide out until your body is parallel to the ground and then rise back up. This sounds much easier than it really is. Break into the movement gradually by performing controlled negatives until you are able to perform the concentric portion properly. Don't allow the hips to sag, the lower back to cave in, or the pelvis to anteriorly rotate. Keep the glutes contracted throughout the movement. If you do not have paper plates or other sliding devices, you can also walk the hands out, with palms flat on the ground.

CORE

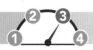
CORE

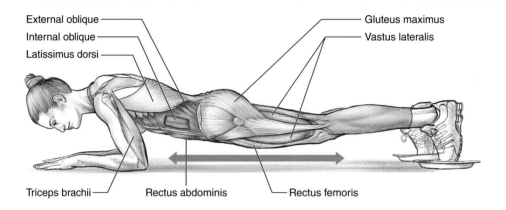

External oblique

Internal oblique

Latissimus dorsi

Gluteus maximus

Vastus lateralis

Triceps brachii

Rectus abdominis

Rectus femoris

Execution

1. Form a pillar by resting your body on the ground and propping your-self on your elbows and feet. Feet are on paper plates. You also can use commercially-available sliding exercise discs or towels on a slick floor.

2. Keep your glutes and quadriceps contracted and your head in a neutral position so your body forms a straight line.

3. Rock the body forward and backward through shoulder flexion and exten-sion. The feet will slide with the forearms serving as a pivot point.

Muscles Involved

Primary: Rectus abdominis, internal oblique, external oblique

Secondary: Gluteus maximus, quadriceps (rectus femoris, vastus lateralis, vastus medialis, vastus intermedius), latissimus dorsi, triceps brachii

Exercise Notes

The sliding body saw is a dynamic variation of the front plank. With your feet on paper plates or another sliding device and your body in a plank position, slide forward and backward to allow your body to pivot around the elbows. Make sure your hips don't sag and that you keep your glutes contracted maximally throughout the movement. Look down to prevent hyperextending the neck. This is a challenging core movement and requires a mastery of other core exercises such as the front plank.

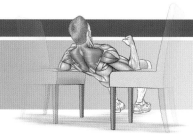

chapter 6

BACK

The back musculature is complex and is vital to producing movement in the human body. All sorts of muscles and connective tissue comprise the back, including the spinal erectors, lats, traps, rhomboids, and the thoracolumbar fascia, which is sometimes called the lumbodorsal fascia. Each muscle plays a pivotal role in producing, reducing, or transferring force from one body segment to another. Before I delve into the functions of the muscles and fascia, I first want to address the importance of a strong back.

Many guys love to train the beach muscles—the pecs, biceps, and abs. Because these muscles reside in the front of the body, they're the most commonly worshipped muscles by gym rats around the world. It's natural to want to build up the beach muscles because there is a perception that everyone admires guys with well-defined pecs, arms, and abdominals. That said, a strong and muscular back is essential for a pleasing physique and a properly functioning body. You won't see wrestlers or football players with wimpy backs. Powerlifters, Olympic weightlifters, and strongmen all have powerful backs as well.

If you think training the back is just for guys, think again. Besides the importance of back strength and stability in sports such as swimming and gymnastics, a well-defined back is a terrific aesthetic asset for women, too. You can't look great in a backless dress or bikini without properly developed back muscles. Having trained hundreds of women during my career as a personal trainer, I can't begin to describe the elation that most women experience when they perform their first full-range pull-up repetition. They're thrilled because most believed that they were not built to be able to bust out a pull-up.

BACK MUSCLES

The latissimus dorsi (lats) is one of the most versatile muscles in the body (figure 6.1). It's responsible for shoulder extension (as in a chin-up), shoulder adduction (as in a down dual-cable pull-down), shoulder internal rotation (turning the arms inward in the shoulder socket), and shoulder transverse abduction (as in a rear delt-raise). They have attachments all over the torso. If you consider the lats' reach through the thoracolumbar fascia, they attach to the vertebrae, pelvis, sacrum, ribs, scapula, and humerus. Moreover, the lats play a role in breathing, stabilizing the lumbar spine, assisting with scapular motion, and transferring forces between the upper and lower body. While all rowing and chinning

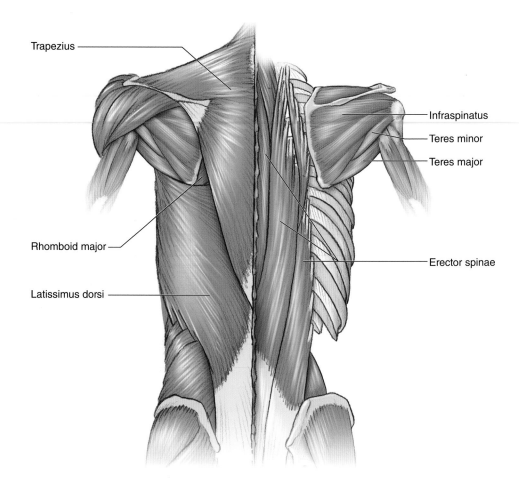

Figure 6.1   Back muscles: trapezius, rhomboid major, latissimus dorsi, infraspinatus, teres minor, teres major, erector spinae.

motions strengthen the lats and scapular muscles, shoulder adduction targets the lower lats to a greater degree, while shoulder extension targets the upper lats and teres major to a greater degree.

Realize, though, that a strong, muscular back isn't solely about having a wide lat spread. To possess an impressive back you need to strengthen all of the muscles that comprise the region. The trapezius muscle is an important shoulder mover and stabilizer. It contains three functional subdivisions, consisting of upper, middle, and lower components. The upper trap fibers are involved in scapular (shoulder blade) elevation and scapular upward rotation and are even involved in neck extension, lateral neck flexion, and neck rotation. The middle trap fibers produce scapular adduction as well as slight scapular elevation and scapular upward rotation. The lower trap fibers are scapular depressors and scapular upward rotators. When the upper and lower trap fibers contract together, they assist the middle fibers in scapular adduction. The rhomboids work in concert with the traps to adduct the scapula, which explains why both muscles are collectively referred to as scapula retractors: They pull the shoulder blades together. The rhomboids are also downward rotators of the scapula.

Development of the spinal erectors (figure 6.2) is critical to long-term lifting prowess. The spinal erectors have many responsibilities. Along with the multifidus they extend the spine, help prevent the spine from flexing (rounding) during deadlifts and squats, and along with muscles such as the quadratus lumborum they laterally flex and rotate the spine.

Last but not least, it is important to mention the role of the thoracolumbar fascia in spinal function. The thoracolumbar fascia (TLF) engulfs the fibers of many core muscles and transfers force between the upper and lower halves of the body. In addition, the TLF, when under tension from certain core muscles such as the lats and glutes, can provide an extension torque on the spine that helps prevent spinal flexion (rounding the low back). Many people are unaware of the lats' role as a stabilizer of the lumbar spine.

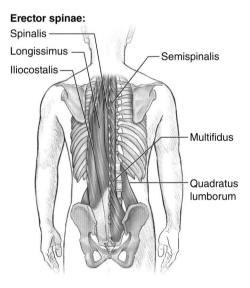

Figure 6.2 Erector spinae, multifidus, quadratus lumborum.

ACTIONS OF THE BACK MUSCLES

The back muscles are involved in nearly every sport action. The spinal erectors are the primary muscles for holding the body in an athletic position, which resembles the positioning of a bent-over row exercise. The spinal erectors are also critical in lifting sports such as powerlifting, Olympic weightlifting, and strongman and in rowing and mixed martial arts. The lats are highly involved in rowing, in addition to gymnastics, swimming, and rock climbing. During sprinting, the opposing pairs of lats and glutes work together to transfer force and keep the body balanced. This diagonal pattern from right lat to left glute and left lat to right glute has been referred to as the *serape effect* by some fitness experts, because of the wrapping action around the body similar to a serape. Furthermore, the lats are heavily involved in throwing, serving, and spiking actions. The traps and rhomboids stabilize the scapula during many athletic motions involving dynamic movement of the upper extremities.

On a personal note, I have not been dealt good genetics for developing impressive back width. Although my back is very thick from many years of deadlifting, I can't achieve the coveted outward flare to my lats no matter how many pull-ups and pull-downs I perform. This is not due to lack of strength either; I'm able to perform chin-ups with an extra 100 pounds (45 kg) attached to a hip belt, and I'm able to deadlift well over 500 pounds (227 kg). An impressive lat flare gives the illusion of a narrower midsection and helps produce an athletic-looking physique, so unfortunately, I'll never appear as aesthetically pleasing as someone with ideal genetics. That said, I have improved my upper-back width considerably through consistent, scientifically based training. I believe that it's wiser to perform only a couple sets of a variety of back exercises than crank out four or more sets of just one or two back exercises. The back contains a lot of muscles and you want maximal development of each muscle to function your best. A variety of back exercises ensures that you leave no stone unturned and dedicate adequate attention to the numerous components of the back musculature.

In chapter 2, I mentioned that your forearms gain strength through the pulling movements. As you progress in pulling strength, your grip will receive a powerful training stimulus. You won't find many people with advanced pull-up and inverted row strength who possess inferior forearm musculature. Get strong and gain endurance through the back exercises listed in this chapter and your entire forearms, both anterior and posterior musculature, will become denser and more muscular.

BACK

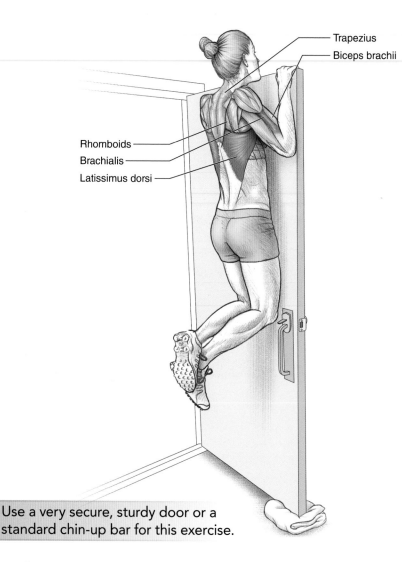

Trapezius

Biceps brachii

Rhomboids

Brachialis

Latissimus dorsi

Safety Tip ▶ Use a very secure, sturdy door or a standard chin-up bar for this exercise.

Execution

1. Place your hands over the top edge of a sturdy door with a pronated grip (palms facing away from the body) and position your body flush against the door. (To keep the door from swinging, wedge a book underneath the door.) Your body is flush against the door at the bottom, but will move away from the door as you rise since the elbows are pined against the door. If a standard chin-up bar is available, that may be the preferred option.

2. Raise your body as high as you can while keeping a straight line from the shoulders to the knees.

3. Lower to starting position and repeat.

Muscles Involved

Primary: Latissimus dorsi, brachialis

Secondary: Trapezius, rhomboids, biceps brachii

Exercise Notes

The pull-up is a challenging movement for the lats, but special consideration needs to be taken to ensure that you do not damage the door, if you choose to use one. I've performed them for years on sturdy doors such as the solid front door of a house with no problems, but because I'm a bigger guy, I'm reluctant to attempt pull-ups on a hollow interior door such as a bathroom or bedroom door. I'm pretty sure I'd pull the door off the hinges! Make sure you perform them off a thick, sturdy door with strong hinges or better yet off a wall. Some exercisers have had success with wedging something such as a big book under a less-sturdy door to reduce the load on the door's hinges, but do this at your own risk; I'd hate for you to damage your property. At any rate, the pull-up has you hinging your body around your elbow joints while your body slides up and down the door, making it even more difficult than a standard chin-up.

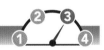

⟨ **VARIATION** ⟩

Rafter Pull-Up

It is important to figure out how to perform pull-ups in your home, and an alternative to the pull-up on a door is the rafter pull-up. Simply grip the top of a smooth, splinter-free rafter with a pronated grip and raise your body as high as it will go. Keep the core tight and don't allow the low back to hyperextend or the pelvis to rotate.

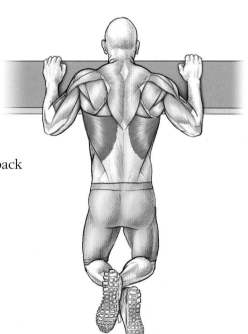

SIDE-TO-SIDE PULL-UP

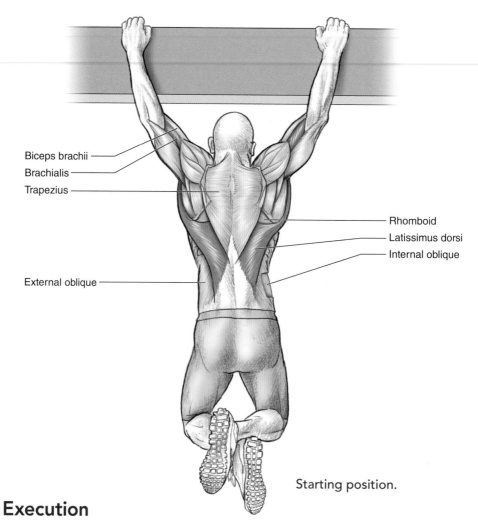

Biceps brachii
Brachialis
Trapezius

Rhomboid
Latissimus dorsi
Internal oblique

External oblique

Starting position.

Execution

1. Hang from a chin-up bar or rafter with the hands pronated and slightly wider than shoulder-width apart. The knees can bend slightly or remain relatively straight.

2. Keeping the chest up and the core tight, pull the body up toward one side until the chin is over the rafter.

3. Lower to starting position and repeat, alternating from side to side.

Muscles Involved

Primary: Latissimus dorsi, brachialis, rectus abdominis

Secondary: Trapezius, rhomboids, biceps brachii, external oblique, internal oblique

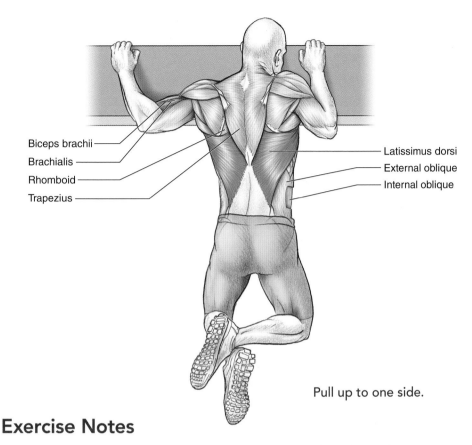

Biceps brachii

Brachialis

Rhomboid

Trapezius

Latissimus dorsi

External oblique

Internal oblique

Pull up to one side.

Exercise Notes

The side-to-side pull-up is an advanced movement that places about 70 percent of the load on the side you're working and 30 percent of the load on the other side. This makes for a more challenging exercise for the lats and other pulling muscles. Keep the core in a neutral position. It will want to contort itself, either hyperextending at the lumbar spine or flexing at the hips. Think of the chin-up as a moving plank (it's good to think this way about push-ups, too) and keep a straight line from the shoulders to the knees throughout the movement.

⟨ VARIATION ⟩

Sliding Side-to-Side Pull-Up

The sliding side-to-side pull-up is a highly advanced maneuver that few people are able to perform. This exercise requires that you first raise the chin over the bar as you would in a standard pull-up. Then slide all the way to one side and all the way to the other side before sliding back to the middle and finally lowering to the starting position. That constitutes one repetition. You won't be able to perform many repetitions of this exercise, assuming you can do it at all.

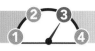
BACK

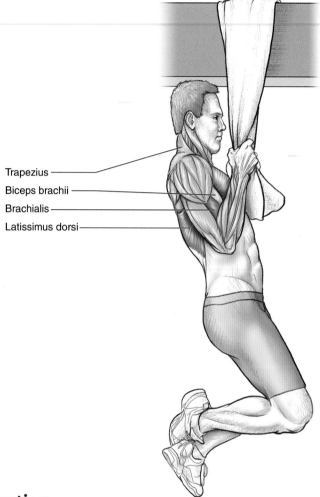

Trapezius
Biceps brachii
Brachialis
Latissimus dorsi

Execution

1. Drape a towel over a chin-up bar or rafter. Grab the towel with both hands.

2. From a stretched position, raise the body while keeping the core in neutral and pulling until the hands meet the upper chest.

3. Lower to starting position and repeat.

Muscles Involved

Primary: Latissimus dorsi, brachialis, forearm muscles such as the flexor carpi radialis and palmaris longus

Secondary: Trapezius, rhomboids, biceps brachii

Exercise Notes

The towel pull-up is an amazing forearm exercise that will build considerable grip strength. Maintain proper pull-up form—don't allow the core to hyperextend, the hips to flex, or the neck to flop. Attempt to spread the towel ends apart at the very top of the motion to maximally engage your scapular retractors. This exercise is needed if you participate in grappling and racket sports, which require maximal grip strength.

⟨ VARIATION ⟩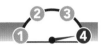

One-Arm Self-Assisted Chin-Up

The one-arm self-assisted chin-up is a highly challenging maneuver that only people with the most advanced upper-body strength will be able to master. However, you can always use the nonworking arm for a bit of assistance, and you just might end up being able to perform an unassisted one-arm chin-up one day. If possible, find a beam narrower than a rafter because this exercise requires a pronated (palms facing away from the body) or supinated (palms facing toward the body) grip. A neutral grip is possible as well if you align your body so you are facing in the same direction as the length of the rafter and hold on to something placed beside the rafter.

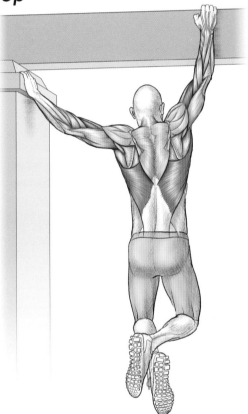

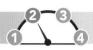

MODIFIED INVERTED ROW

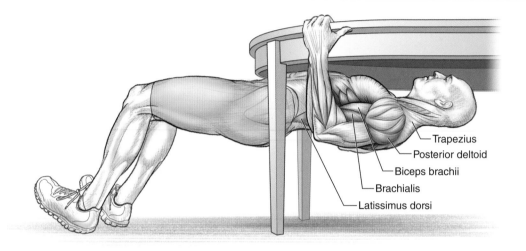

Trapezius
Posterior deltoid
Biceps brachii
Brachialis
Latissimus dorsi

Execution

1. Grasp the sides of a sturdy table, keeping the knees bent at about 90-135 degrees and heels planted firmly on the ground. It's a good idea to perform this exercise over a forgiving surface such as soft carpeting.

2. Keeping the body in a straight line from the knees to the shoulders, pull your body up until your chest meets the table.

3. Lower your body to starting position under control.

Muscles Involved

Primary: Latissimus dorsi, brachialis, posterior deltoid
Secondary: Trapezius, rhomboids, biceps brachii

Exercise Notes

The inverted row is a staple upper-body pulling movement using body weight. If you don't have access to a standard exercise bar or suspension system, it can be performed several ways. First, if you have a table that is the right width and doesn't have anything blocking your path, you can use a table by holding on to the sides. Second, if you have a sturdy broomstick, you can suspend it between two chairs and use it as a rowing bar. Third, you can use the edges of two chairs by positioning the arms close to the end of the chairs and wrapping the hands over the top in a neutral position. Make sure you keep the chest up and use a full range of motion on these. When you gain proficiency, you can elevate your feet on a chair to increase the exercise's difficulty. The steeper the angle, the easier the exercise. The most challenging angle of performance is achieved when the body is parallel to the ground.

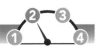
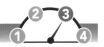

⟨ VARIATION ⟩

Feet-Elevated Inverted Row

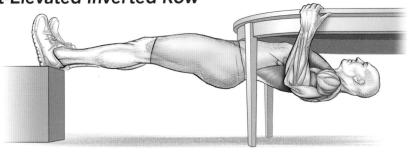

Once you reach proficiency with the modified inverted row, you can make the movement more challenging by progressing to the feet-elevated variation. Remember to keep the body in a straight line and squeeze the shoulder blades together at the top position.

⟨ VARIATION ⟩

Towel Inverted Row

The towel inverted row is another option. You'll likely be able to figure out a way to drape a towel over a table, the corner of a table, two tall chairs, or even a door if you have a very long towel. You can get an efficient workout while positioning the body at a steeper incline. Focus on keeping the elbows to the sides and the chest high, and squeeze the shoulder blades back and down.

BACK

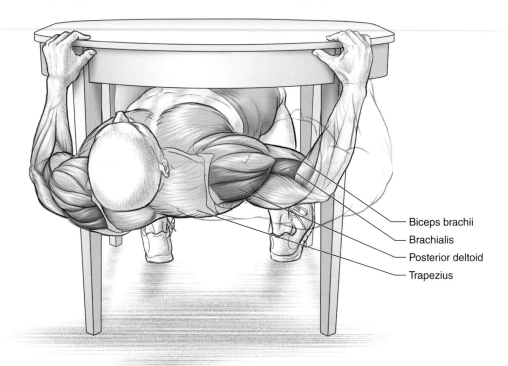

Biceps brachii
Brachialis
Posterior deltoid
Trapezius

Execution

1. Begin suspended in a stretched position with the body in a straight line and the core tight with legs straight, heels against the ground, and palms facing forward.
2. Raise the body to one side.
3. Lower the body to the starting position and repeat, alternating sides.

Muscles Involved

Primary: Latissimus dorsi, brachialis, posterior deltoid
Secondary: Trapezius, rhomboids, biceps brachii

Exercise Notes

The side-to-side inverted row is an advanced movement, and just like the side-to-side pull-up, it places about 70 percent of the load on the side you're working and 30 percent of the load on the other side. This makes for a much more challenging exercise for the lats and scapular muscles. Rowing strength is critical for long-term shoulder health, so don't underestimate its importance. Although they're not as sexy as pull-ups, they're every bit as important for scapular stability and shoulder health.

⟨ VARIATION ⟩

Sliding Side-to-Side Inverted Row

The sliding side-to-side inverted row is a highly advanced maneuver. As in the case of the sliding side-to-side pull-up, not many people will be able to perform this exercise right off the bat. If possible start with the body at a steep incline so you learn how to perform the movement correctly because it's easy to waste energy trying to keep the body stable through compensatory rotary motion or body contortion. From a relaxed position, row the body straight up, then slide the body all the way to one side, then all the way to the other side, then back to the middle, and finally back down. Congratulations, you just performed one repetition. Alternate the side you shift to first on each repetition.

⟨ VARIATION ⟩

One-Arm Inverted Row

Once you've mastered the two-arm row variations, it's time to start practicing one-arm inverted rows. If you can start with a substantial body incline you'll be able to perform the movement with good form right off the bat. It's okay to rotate a little bit at first, but over time try to limit rotation throughout the movement. This exercise is well suited for using a towel.

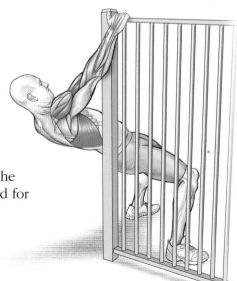

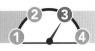

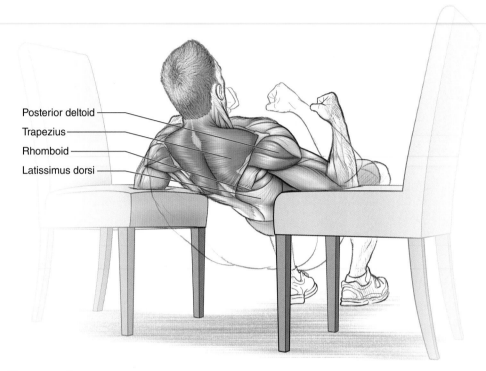

BACK

Posterior deltoid

Trapezius

Rhomboid

Latissimus dorsi

Execution

1. Position your body between two couches, chairs, or weight benches with the feet on the floor, the hips extended in line with the shoulders, and the backs of the upper arms resting on the platform at about 45-degree angles relative to the torso.

2. Dig your elbows into the platform and squeeze your shoulder blades together. This will cause your chest to rise in a short range of motion.

3. Lower the body to starting position under control and repeat.

Muscles Involved

Primary: Trapezius, rhomboids, posterior deltoid

Secondary: Latissimus dorsi, gluteus maximus, quadriceps (rectus femoris, vastus lateralis, vastus medialis, vastus intermedius), erector spinae (spinalis, longissimus, iliocostalis), hamstrings (biceps femoris, semitendinosus, semimembranosus)

Exercise Notes

During this exercise you hold your body in a bridging motion while suspended between two chairs. By digging your elbows into the chairs and squeezing the scapulae together you'll perform a short-range movement that targets the scapula retractors. Keep the chest up and the hips high, and control the movement on the way down.

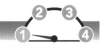
⟨ **VARIATION** ⟩

Corner Scapular Shrug

Stand with your back to a corner and the upper arms in position against the two walls and the feet a few feet out in front of the corner. Move the body outward, away from the corner, by squeezing the scapulae together. This is a short-range movement that targets the scapula retractors. Adjust your foot position to find the appropriate distance that creates just the right challenge.

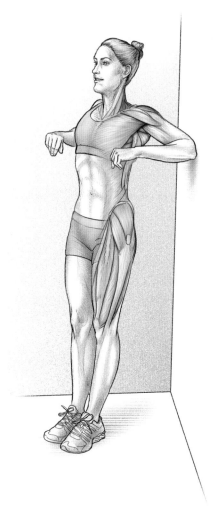

BACK

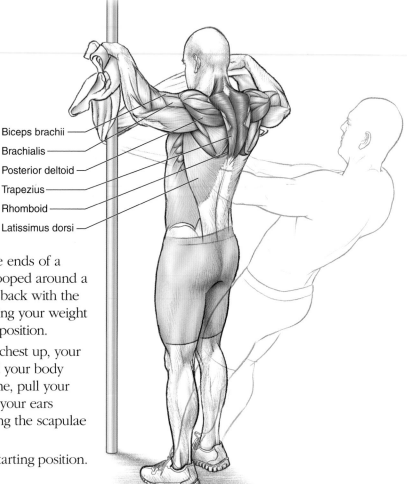

Biceps brachii

Brachialis

Posterior deltoid

Trapezius

Rhomboid

Latissimus dorsi

Execution

1. Hold on to the ends of a towel that is looped around a pole and lean back with the towel supporting your weight in a stretched position.

2. Keeping your chest up, your core tight, and your body in a straight line, pull your hands toward your ears while squeezing the scapulae together.

3. Lower to the starting position.

Muscles Involved

Primary: Trapezius, rhomboids, posterior deltoid

Secondary: Latissimus dorsi, brachialis, biceps brachii

Exercise Notes

The towel face pull is an excellent exercise to perform from time to time to develop scapular stability and shoulder health. It works the scapular muscles slightly differently than rowing movements and provides variety. You won't be able to perform towel face pulls from the same angle that you perform inverted rows because you won't be quite as strong in this movement pattern and will therefore require a steeper body angle. Keep the chest up and use a full range of motion. This exercise doesn't require much of an angle to challenge the muscles if you keep the body tight and squeeze the scapula together at the end range.

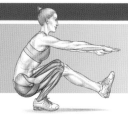

chapter 7

THIGHS

Go to any gym and you'll see that well-developed upper bodies are a dime a dozen. Even folks who train with just their own body weight typically have impressive pecs, shoulders, lats, and arms. But most of these lifters suffer from light bulb syndrome, with legs befitting a chicken. Many lifters slave away working their upper bodies only to skip leg training or, at best, perform a couple of token sets of leg presses, leg extensions, and leg curls on leg day. While much better than avoiding leg training altogether and leaps and bounds above claiming to hit the legs by running on the treadmill, this abbreviated leg workout leaves much room for improvement. And as I mentioned before, effective upper-body training with just body weight is intuitive for many lifters because most exercisers are well aware of push-ups, pull-ups, and sit-ups, but most don't have the slightest clue how to work the legs effectively with just their body weight. The good news is that with a little ingenuity, it's easy to develop impressive lower-body musculature using just the weight of one's own body for resistance.

I'm very proud of my leg development because it's indicative of many years of hard work. Not that I'm genetically predisposed to having muscular thighs, far from it. But through many years of consistency and effort I've built them up to appreciable levels. And although I train with weights, I'm certain that I could maintain my thigh musculature, and quite possibly build on it, by switching solely to bodyweight training for the lower body. How can I be so sure? Because as you'll soon see, there are dozens of challenging and effective bodyweight exercises for the legs.

Lifters need to take pride in their lower body development and learn to appreciate the challenges associated with lower-body training. After years of trying, I finally convinced my stepbrother to start training his legs. Previously he worked his chest and arms twice a week and his back and shoulders twice a week and did no leg training whatsoever. I coerced him into adding one leg day a week and he remarked that "the leg day is just as hard as all the upper-body days combined." He's right; upper-body exercises just don't tax you like compound lower-body exercises, primarily because of the enormous amount of muscle mass being worked during the set. For example, a Bulgarian split squat will involve the quadriceps, gluteus maximus, and hamstrings as prime movers, but many other muscles also contribute to the movement including the gastrocnemius, soleus, adductors, gluteus medius, gluteus minimus, quadratus lumborum, and multifidus.

Leg training for women is an absolute must. Athletic-looking thighs greatly enhance the appearance when wearing jeans, a skirt or dress, a bathing suit, or nothing at all. But lower-body training isn't just for developing shape. Because these exercises target the most muscle mass, they require a considerable amount of energy to perform and therefore are terrific for shedding body fat. In fact, a hardcore leg workout does more for bringing out the abs than traditional core exercises. And while you're training your legs, you're creating a metabolic afterburn that keeps the engines revved for more than 24 hours following the actual workout. Ultimately, you'll burn extra calories around the clock, helping to keep you lean all over.

THIGH MUSCLES

Many muscles comprise the thigh. The thigh muscles many people think of first are the quadriceps and the hamstrings. You have four quadriceps muscles: the rectus femoris (which is also a hip flexor), vastus intermedius, vastus lateralis, and vastus medialis (figure 7.1a). Their job is to extend the knee joint. You have three hamstring muscles: the biceps femoris, semitendinosus, and semimembranosus (figure 7.1b). Their job is to extend the hip and flex the knee. The biceps femoris has a long head and a short head. The short head is the only hamstring muscle that doesn't cross the hip joint and therefore doesn't extend the hip.

You also have the adductor group consisting of the adductor longus, adductor brevis, and adductor magnus. These muscles make up a considerable portion of the thigh and shouldn't be neglected. While their primary role is adduction (moving the leg toward the center of the body), they also contribute to hip flexion and hip extension, especially the hamstring portion of the adductor magnus, depending on the position of the thigh. Lucky for you, the adductors receive a good training stimulus during single-leg exercises.

There are plenty of other thigh muscles, including the psoas (an important hip flexor), gracilis, pectineus, and sartorius, but it's not mandatory for you to know every muscle's precise function. It is, however, mandatory that you understand how to effectively train the legs with proper form.

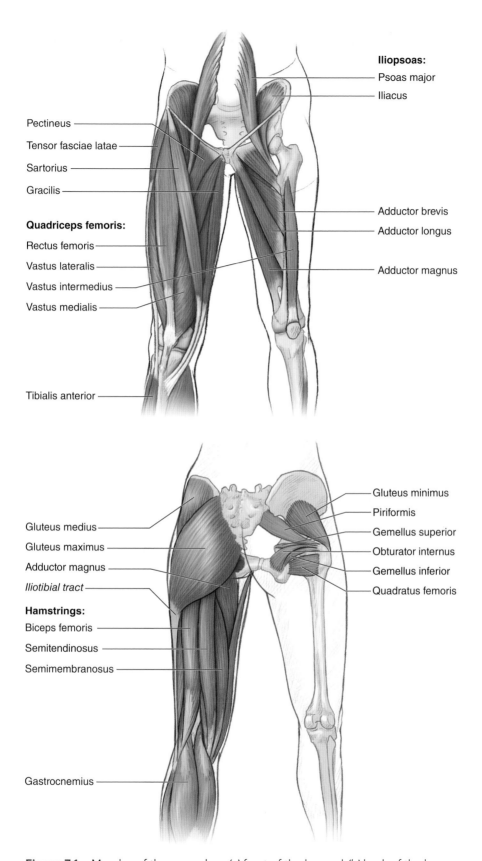

Figure 7.1 Muscles of the upper leg: *(a)* front of the leg and *(b)* back of the leg.

THIGH ACTIONS AND MOVEMENTS

The thigh muscles are heavily involved in sports and functional movement. The quadriceps might be the most important muscles in vertical jumping, and they're critical for running, cutting, landing, and decelerating as well. The hamstrings might be the most important muscles in sprint running. In weight training, the quadriceps contribute considerably to the squat exercise and the hamstrings contribute considerably to the deadlift exercise. I will be unable to name every sport action that requires ample leg strength and power; there are simply too many to mention. Every ground sport that requires speed, power, and agility relies predominantly on the leg muscles, and even swimming, rowing, and climbing uses combined hip and knee extension for propulsion. Because the hamstrings cross both the knee and hip joints, they play critical roles in transferring power from the knee joint to the hip joint during explosive movement. Considering that most sports are performed one leg at a time, it makes sense to include plenty of single-leg lower-body exercises in your routine. Single-leg exercises develop sensorimotor (balance) skills while simultaneously improving strength and power.

Many athletes are considered quad dominant because their quadriceps overpower their hamstrings. Athletes with overpowered quadriceps in relation to the hamstrings typically fail to move ideally when jumping, running, landing, and cutting, thereby predisposing themselves to injury. For this reason it's important to develop strong hamstrings. Possessing strong quadriceps is important for sports, but you should also possess strong hamstrings as both hip extensors and knee flexors. Knee-flexion exercises work more on the distal part of the hamstrings (the part closer to the knees), while hip-extension exercises work more on the proximal part of the hamstrings (the part closer to the hips). This chapter includes a variety of hamstring exercises so you can strengthen them through all of their roles and through full ranges of motion, leaving you with no weaknesses.

Many of the movement patterns described in this chapter lay the foundation for your athletic success. The fundamental motor patterns involved in bodyweight squatting, bending (hip hinging), lunging, and bridging play a big role in determining how you move, how you transfer loading, and how you absorb shock during high-force or high-velocity sport actions. For this reason, master the basics and learn proper form before moving on to more challenging exercise variations.

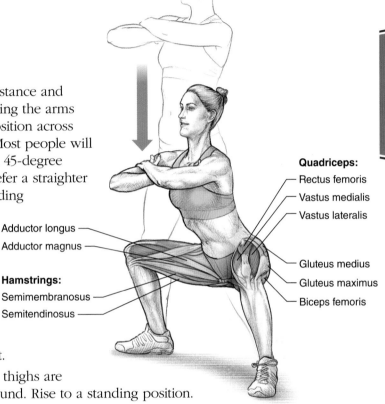

Execution

1. Take a very wide stance and flare the feet, placing the arms in the mummy position across the upper body. Most people will gravitate toward a 45-degree flare but some prefer a straighter foot angle, depending on their hip anatomy.

2. Squat by sitting back, keeping the trunk upright and knees forced outward throughout the movement.

3. Descend until the thighs are parallel to the ground. Rise to a standing position.

Adductor longus
Adductor magnus

Hamstrings:
Semimembranosus
Semitendinosus

Quadriceps:
Rectus femoris
Vastus medialis
Vastus lateralis

Gluteus medius
Gluteus maximus
Biceps femoris

Muscles Involved

Primary: Quadriceps (rectus femoris, vastus lateralis, vastus medialis, vastus intermedius)

Secondary: Gluteus maximus, gluteus medius, gluteus minimus, hamstrings (biceps femoris, semitendinosus, semimembranosus), adductor magnus, adductor longus, adductor brevis, erector spinae (spinalis, longissimus, iliocostalis), deep-hip external rotators

Exercise Notes

The sumo squat is an excellent exercise because it teaches you to squat using more than just the quadriceps. In this case, the hip adductors and abductors come into play more because of the biomechanics of the exercise. Keep the chest up and get a nice stretch in the hip extensors at the bottom of the movement.

WALL SQUAT ISOHOLD

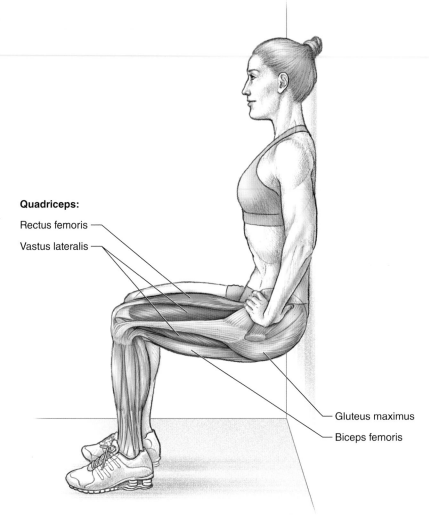

Quadriceps:

Rectus femoris

Vastus lateralis

Gluteus maximus

Biceps femoris

Execution

1. Lean your back against a wall with your feet in front of you, hands on the hips.

2. Lower the body until the hips reach a 90-degree angle and the thighs are parallel to the ground. The knees are at a 90-degree angle with the shins perpendicular to the ground and the feet flat on the ground.

3. Hold for the desired amount of time: 30 seconds for beginners up to 120 seconds for advanced.

Muscles Involved

Primary: Quadriceps (rectus femoris, vastus lateralis, vastus medialis, vastus intermedius)

Secondary: Gluteus maximus, hamstrings (biceps femoris, semitendinosus, semimembranosus)

Exercise Notes

The wall squat isohold serves as a fundamental quadriceps endurance exercise. You can perform it anywhere you find a wall. Keep perfect posture throughout the duration of the set by keeping the chest up and sitting tall. Add variety to this exercise by changing the hip angle during the set. For example, start at a more difficult hip angle that places your hips lower than your knees, then move to a thigh-parallel position as the set gets challenging, and finally moving to a hips-higher-than-knees position.

⟨ VARIATION ⟩

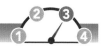

Wall Squat March

Once the wall squat isohold becomes easy, make the exercise more challenging by performing marches. You'll probably need to start with the hips higher than the knees because this is not an easy variation. Over time you should be able to perform the movement from a 90-degree hip angle. Simply raise one leg off the ground and hold for time, then switch to the other leg. Hold for time, then switch to the other leg. Alternate from one leg to the other several times to fatigue the quadriceps.

BOX SQUAT

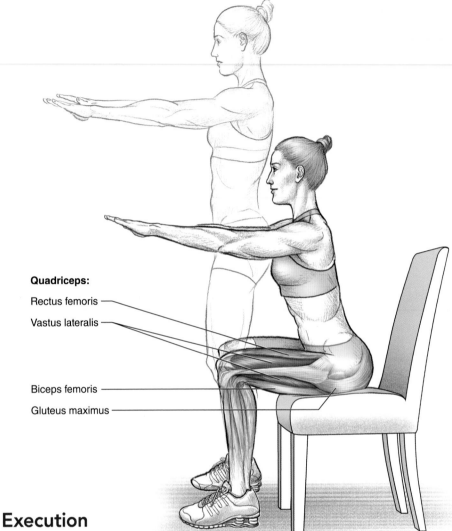

Quadriceps:

Rectus femoris

Vastus lateralis

Biceps femoris

Gluteus maximus

Execution

1. Stand with your feet wider than shoulder-width apart and the feet flared to your preference. Stand very close to the edge of a sturdy box, bench, chair, step, or stool.

2. Initiate the movement by breaking at the hips and sitting back, keeping the chest up, the knees out so they track over the toes, and the shins perpendicular to the floor. Remember to push through the heels.

3. Pause for a moment while sitting on the box and then rise, making sure to squeeze the glutes to lockout.

Muscles Involved

Primary: Quadriceps (rectus femoris, vastus lateralis, vastus medialis, vastus intermedius)

Secondary: Gluteus maximus, gluteus medius, gluteus minimus, hamstrings (biceps femoris, semitendinosus, semimembranosus), erector spinae (spinalis, longissimus, iliocostalis)

Exercise Notes

The box squat is the fundamental squat pattern you should master before attempting other types of squats. This squat pattern teaches you how to sit back and use your hips. It also teaches you to keep the knees out to prevent them from caving in during the movement. Keep your chest up and push through your heels throughout the movement. Most people can start with a box height that puts their thighs parallel to the ground when seated. Less-fit people need to start with a box that's a bit higher, and athletic folks will be able to go right to the low box squat. It is critical that you learn how to use the hips while squatting because this practice will transfer to jumping and agility performance on the field, which will spare the knees and allow for greater explosiveness.

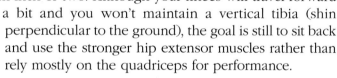

Low Box Squat

The low box squat is performed with a sturdy box that is about 12 inches (30 cm) high, give or take an inch or two. Although your knees will travel forward a bit and you won't maintain a vertical tibia (shin perpendicular to the ground), the goal is still to sit back and use the stronger hip extensor muscles rather than rely mostly on the quadriceps for performance.

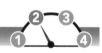

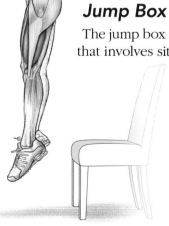

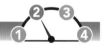

Jump Box Squat

The jump box squat is an explosive plyometric variation that involves sitting back on to the box (or sturdy chair) as you would in a typical box squat and then forcefully rising into a jump. Land softly and absorb shock properly by distributing the load among all the joints at play, especially the hips.

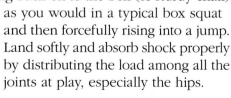

FULL SQUAT

Execution

1. Stand with a narrow stance and feet flared. Most people find a 30-degree foot flare most comfortable, but this depends on individual hip anatomy. Place the hands in a mummy position, crossed in front of the body.

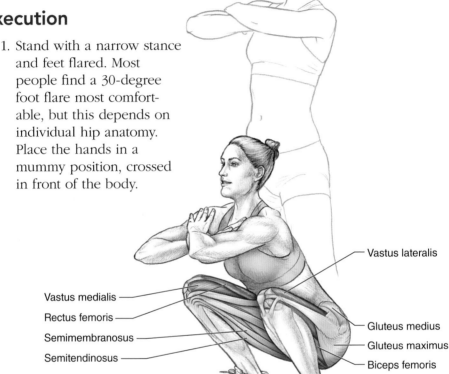

Vastus lateralis

Vastus medialis

Rectus femoris

Semimembranosus

Semitendinosus

Gluteus medius

Gluteus maximus

Biceps femoris

2. Initiate the movement by simultaneously breaking at the knees and hips and dropping straight down. Keep the weight on the whole foot, keep the chest up, and force the knees out of the bottom of the movement so that the knees track over the middle of the feet.

3. Descend as deeply as possible while keeping a flat lower back. Rise to a standing position.

Muscles Involved

Primary: Quadriceps (rectus femoris, vastus lateralis, vastus medialis, vastus intermedius)

Secondary: Gluteus maximus, gluteus medius, gluteus minimus, hamstrings (biceps femoris, semitendinosus, semimembranosus), erector spinae (spinalis, longissimus, iliocostalis)

Exercise Notes

The full squat is a seemingly simple exercise but it actually requires considerable ankle dorsiflexion flexibility, hip flexion flexibility, and thoracic extension flexibility. This means that your knees have to be able to travel forward pretty far at the bottom of the movement without rising onto the toes, the hips need to be able to sink low with no rounding of the low back or tucking of the pelvis, and the upper back needs to stay tight to prevent upper-back rounding. For this reason, many people find that they cannot perform this movement until they increase their mobility. The full squat also requires sufficient core stability and glute activation, so be patient and focus on quality not quantity. As time goes on, full squats will become easier, but take your time working into them and building the requisite flexibility and stability to perform the movement correctly. The hips will sink between the knees, which are forced outward during a proper full squat.

⟨ VARIATION ⟩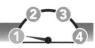

Counterbalance Full Squat

People who struggle with full squats can raise their arms as the squat descends, thereby creating a counterbalance effect that shifts emphasis away from the weaker knee joint and toward the stronger hip joint. Simply flex the shoulders and lift the arms until they are parallel to the ground as the hips flex during the descent of the squat movement.

⟨ VARIATION ⟩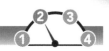

Jump Full Squat

When the full squat becomes too easy, increase the challenge to the thigh musculature by rising forcefully into a jump. Remember to squat all the way down because this is not a standard vertical jump. Squat, keep the chest up and knees out, jump as high as possible, and then use the hips to absorb the landing.

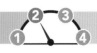
THIGHS

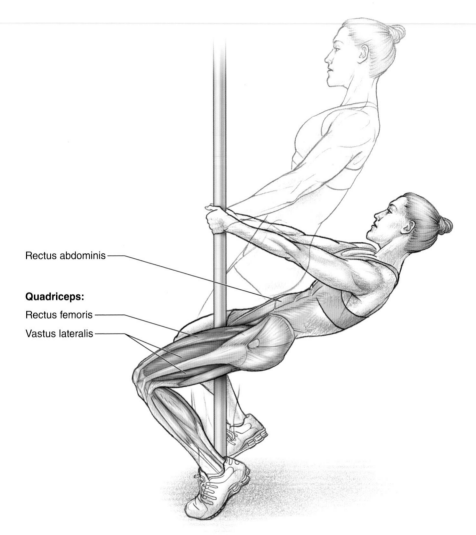

Rectus abdominis

Quadriceps:

Rectus femoris

Vastus lateralis

Execution

1. Begin in a standing position with a narrow stance. Grasp something in front of you for balance.

2. Descend by breaking at the knees and shifting them forward while leaning the torso back and rising onto the toes.

3. Descend until the desired depth is reached and then rise to return to starting position.

Muscles Involved

Primary: Quadriceps (rectus femoris, vastus lateralis, vastus medialis, vastus intermedius)

Secondary: Rectus abdominis

Exercise Notes

The sissy squat can be thought of as a bodyweight leg extension because it targets the quadriceps and eliminates hip extensor involvement. Many people find this exercise problematic because it puts considerable pressure on the knee joint, so play it safe and ease your way into this exercise. Descend only to a depth that feels comfortable in the knees and gradually increase the depth over time. Attempt to feel the quadriceps controlling the movement throughout the set.

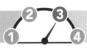
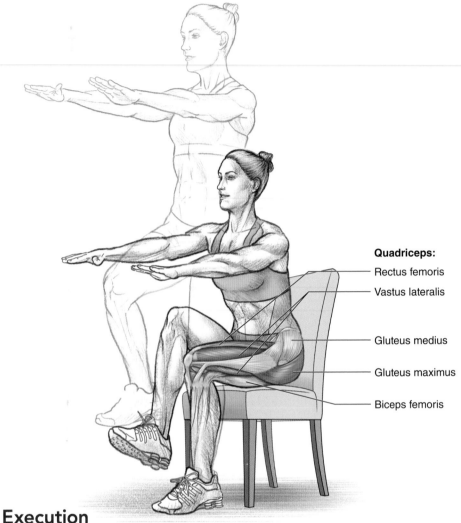

Quadriceps:
Rectus femoris
Vastus lateralis

Gluteus medius

Gluteus maximus

Biceps femoris

Execution

1. Stand in front of a sturdy box, bench, chair, step, or stool, with the hands in front of the body.

2. Standing on one leg, sit back and down onto the surface, keeping the chest up and the spine rigid. The knee tracks over the midfoot as you push through the heel.

3. Lift the arms for counterbalance. Pause on the box for a moment, then rise to return to starting position, making sure to squeeze the glutes.

Muscles Involved

Primary: Quadriceps (rectus femoris, vastus lateralis, vastus medialis, vastus intermedius), gluteus maximus

Secondary: Hamstrings (biceps femoris, semitendinosus, semimembranosus), adductor magnus, adductor longus, adductor brevis, gluteus medius, gluteus minimus, deep-hip external rotators

Exercise Notes

The single-leg box squat is an effective single-leg movement that allows you to adjust for difficulty by simply changing the height of the box. Beginners need to master the double-leg version before moving on to the single-leg version. Once proficiency in the double-leg pattern is reached, begin performing the single-leg version with a high box to allow you to learn proper technique. Don't let your knee cave in or out. Raising the arms during the movement serves as an effective countermovement, shifting the burden away from the knees and onto the hips.

⟨ **VARIATION** ⟩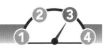

Single-Leg Low-Box Squat

As you progress in the single-leg box squat, you'll be able to reduce the height of the box to continue increasing the exercise's effectiveness. As you move to lower box heights, you won't be able to sit back quite as far and you'll need to allow the knee to travel forward a bit to maintain balance. Keep the low back arched and contract the spinal erectors forcefully to keep the pelvis from tucking under.

⟨ **VARIATION** ⟩

Jumping Single-Leg Box Squat

The jumping single-leg box squat is an advanced movement that requires considerable hip stability, balance, and strength. Simply add a jump to the movement by accelerating the body upward during the concentric phase with enough power to leave the ground, and make sure that the jump appears fluid and natural. If it's not, you're not yet ready for this variation. Single-leg movements challenge the body's sensorimotor skills, promoting improvements in balance that are critical, especially as you age.

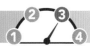

SKATER SQUAT

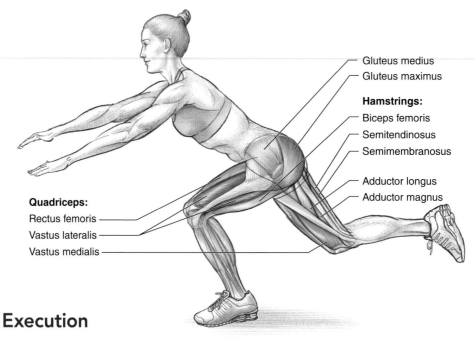

Gluteus medius
Gluteus maximus

Hamstrings:
Biceps femoris
Semitendinosus
Semimembranosus

Adductor longus
Adductor magnus

Quadriceps:
Rectus femoris
Vastus lateralis
Vastus medialis

Execution

1. Stand on one foot and place the hands in front of the body.
2. Sit back and down, breaking at the hips and knees while leaning forward at the trunk.
3. Descend until the knee of the nonworking leg approaches or touches the ground. Stand up to return to starting position. Perform all the repetitions with the weaker leg first and then switch and repeat with the stronger leg.

Muscles Involved

Primary: Quadriceps (rectus femoris, vastus lateralis, vastus medialis, vastus intermedius), gluteus maximus

Secondary: Hamstrings (biceps femoris, semitendinosus, semimembranosus), adductor magnus, adductor longus, adductor brevis, gluteus medius, gluteus minimus, deep-hip external rotators

Exercise Notes

The skater squat is a phenomenal lower-body exercise that works the thighs and hips thoroughly. Flex the shoulders to provide counterbalance and lower yourself all the way until the back knee touches or skims the ground. You can place a pillow or towel on the ground so the knee doesn't smash into the floor.

Because most sports are played on one leg at a time, it makes sense to include a lot of single-leg exercises in your regimen. In general, single-leg exercises challenge the lateral and rotary stability of the hips and require coordination of muscles such as the hip adductors, hip abductors, hip rotators, quadratus lumborum, and multifidus to prevent lateral shifting or twisting during the movement.

⟨ **VARIATION** ⟩

Skater Squat With Knee Raise

Adding a knee raise further challenges your single-leg stability because you'll be standing on one leg the entire time, taking the nonworking leg from a position of hip extension to hip flexion. Squeeze the glute of the working leg and stand tall when the hip of the free leg is at its highest point of flexion.

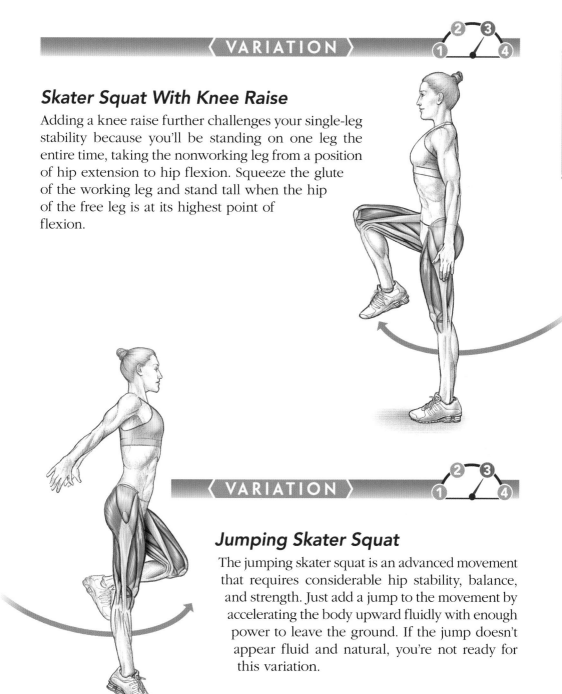

⟨ **VARIATION** ⟩

Jumping Skater Squat

The jumping skater squat is an advanced movement that requires considerable hip stability, balance, and strength. Just add a jump to the movement by accelerating the body upward fluidly with enough power to leave the ground. If the jump doesn't appear fluid and natural, you're not ready for this variation.

STATIC LUNGE

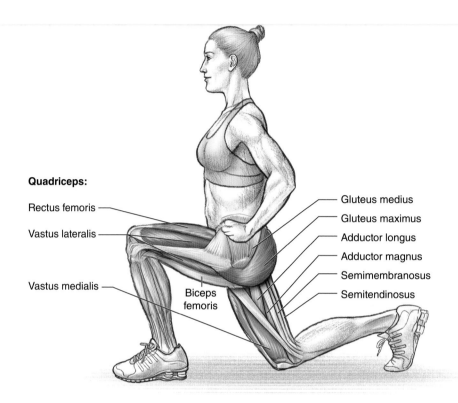

Quadriceps:

Rectus femoris

Vastus lateralis

Vastus medialis

Biceps femoris

Gluteus medius

Gluteus maximus

Adductor longus

Adductor magnus

Semimembranosus

Semitendinosus

Execution

1. Get in a split-stance position that is wide enough that your front shin is vertical at the bottom of the lunge. Your hands are on the hips and feet pointed straight ahead.

2. Keeping the torso upright, descend until the back knee approaches or touches the ground.

3. Return to starting position.

Muscles Involved

Primary: Quadriceps (rectus femoris, vastus lateralis, vastus medialis, vastus intermedius), gluteus maximus

Secondary: Hamstrings (biceps femoris, semitendinosus, semimembranosus), adductor magnus, adductor longus, adductor brevis, gluteus medius, gluteus minimus, deep-hip external rotators

motion and torque loading on the hips. Try to feel the glute of the front leg absorbing the force and helping to spring the body back into position.

Many people fail to step back with a long enough stride. There's a sweet spot in terms of stride length that maximizes the exercise's effectiveness. In time you'll learn the perfect distance.

Lunges are well known for their ability to create sore glutes and sore adductors. The adductor magnus in particular gets hammered during this movement because down low the adductors are excellent hip extensors.

‹ VARIATION ›

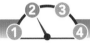

Deficit Reverse Lunge

Once you master the reverse lunge, you can increase the exercise's difficulty by standing on a step, sturdy box, or short table that is approximately 6 to 10 inches (15-25 cm) high. The same rules apply, but this variation will increase your hip range of motion and provide a greater stretch to the working glute. Beware the following day. This exercise may impair your ability to sit down without appearing like an old man or woman. In other words, the stretch loading on the hips can produce serious glute soreness.

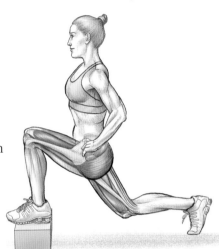

‹ VARIATION ›

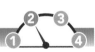

Step-Up and Reverse Lunge Hybrid

The step-up and reverse lunge hybrid is one of my favorite exercises. Once you've mastered the step-up and deficit reverse lunge, you can perform a combination lift that is highly effective. Stand on top of the step, making sure your entire foot is on the step so you can push through the heel. Step back and upon landing, sink into a lunge position, feeling a big stretch in the glute. Keeping the chest up and a slight forward lean, spring up. Try to keep most of the emphasis on the front leg and avoid using the back leg for too much assistance.

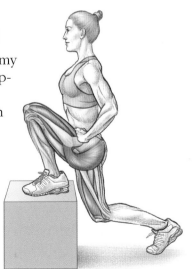

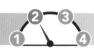

THIGHS

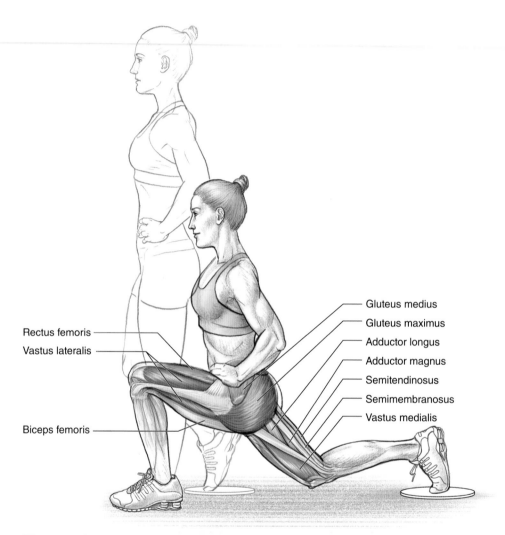

Rectus femoris
Vastus lateralis

Biceps femoris

Gluteus medius
Gluteus maximus
Adductor longus
Adductor magnus
Semitendinosus
Semimembranosus
Vastus medialis

Execution

1. Stand with feet pointed straight ahead about shoulder-width apart with hands on the hips and one foot on a paper plate. You also may use a commercially-available sliding exercise disc or, on a slick floor, a small hand towel.

2. Keeping most of the weight on the foot that isn't on the plate, slide the foot on the plate back and lean forward to an approximately 30-degree trunk angle, sinking into the working hip and descending until the back knee approaches or touches the ground.

3. Rise to starting position.

Muscles Involved

Primary: Quadriceps (rectus femoris, vastus lateralis, vastus medialis, vastus intermedius), gluteus maximus

Secondary: Hamstrings (biceps femoris, semitendinosus, semimembranosus), adductor magnus, adductor longus, adductor brevis, gluteus medius, gluteus minimus, deep-hip external rotators

Exercise Notes

This is similar to the reverse lunge, except that in the sliding lunge your foot always maintains contact with the ground. Many people prefer this variation over the reverse lunge, but it's up to the individual. I like the standard reverse lunge better, but give them both a try and judge for yourself. At any rate, both are great variations and the lunge pattern is an essential pattern for comprehensive hip strength, so you can't go wrong by performing both variations from time to time.

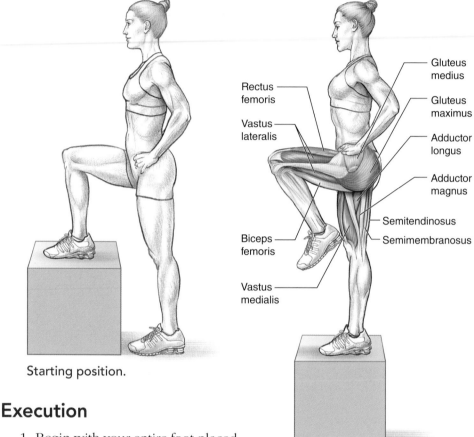

Rectus femoris

Vastus lateralis

Biceps femoris

Vastus medialis

Gluteus medius

Gluteus maximus

Adductor longus

Adductor magnus

Semitendinosus

Semimembranosus

Starting position.

Execution

1. Begin with your entire foot placed on top of a step, sturdy box, chair, or weight bench. The other foot remains on the ground.

2. Shift your weight forward and lift your body weight by stepping up, making sure that the top leg does most of the work and the bottom leg doesn't provide too much momentum.

3. Stand tall and squeeze the working glute. Do not touch the working leg to the bench and swing the nongrounded knee upward by flexing the hip. Lower yourself slowly and under control back to starting position.

Muscles Involved

Primary: Quadriceps (rectus femoris, vastus lateralis, vastus medialis, vastus intermedius), gluteus maximus

Secondary: Hamstrings (biceps femoris, semitendinosus, semimembranosus), adductor magnus, adductor longus, adductor brevis, gluteus medius, gluteus minimus, deep-hip external rotators, psoas

Exercise Notes

The step-up is a classic exercise that has stood the test of time. Weaker people must start from a very low height and work their way up to greater heights over time. Do not make the mistake of placing just half of your foot on the step because this prevents you from pushing through your heel. Furthermore, do not use the bottom leg to help blast yourself up, which prevents you from relying predominantly on the working leg. Finally, do not touch the foot of the free leg on the box as you rise. This encourages you to catch yourself in a quarter-squat position and use both legs to complete the movement. Use a full range of motion and make the intended leg do most of the work from start to finish.

⟨ VARIATION ⟩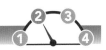

High Step-Up

As you gain proficiency in the standard step-up, increase the difficulty of the exercise by continuing to find higher steps. Never go so high that you can't maintain an arch in the low back and the pelvis in a neutral position or slightly tilted back. Do not let the lower back round or the pelvis tuck under. Going ultrahigh encourages lumbar flexion and posterior pelvic tilt, which you should avoid. This variation is a favorite glute exercise of many of my female clients and, when performed correctly, provides an excellent single-leg strengthening stimulus.

⟨ VARIATION ⟩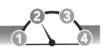

Alternating Jump Step-Up

Perform a plyometric style of step-up by adding an explosive step-up and then jumping from one side of the step to the other in an alternating fashion. Aim to achieve maximum height on the jump and make sure your posture stays solid throughout the set.

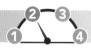
THIGHS

Execution

1. Stand in front of a step, stair, couch, bed, table, stool, or weight bench. Reach back with one foot, resting the top of the foot on the top of the surface. (Think laces down.)

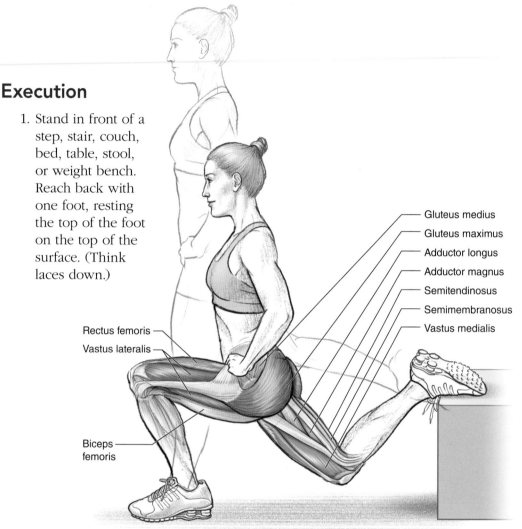

Gluteus medius

Gluteus maximus

Adductor longus

Adductor magnus

Semitendinosus

Semimembranosus

Vastus medialis

Rectus femoris

Vastus lateralis

Biceps femoris

2. With an upright trunk or a slight forward lean, sink the knee of the rear leg down and slightly back while trying to keep most of the body weight on the front leg.

3. Descend until the back knee almost touches or touches the ground. Rise to starting position.

Muscles Involved

Primary: Quadriceps (rectus femoris, vastus lateralis, vastus medialis, vastus intermedius), gluteus maximus

Secondary: Hamstrings (biceps femoris, semitendinosus, semimembranosus), adductor magnus, adductor longus, adductor brevis, gluteus medius, gluteus minimus, deep-hip external rotators

Exercise Notes

The Bulgarian split squat has gained popularity over the past decade and is indeed an amazing exercise. Many people struggle to find the optimal stride length. Typically it's longer than most people think, but you don't want too big a stride. The knee of the front leg will not move past the toes if you perform this movement properly because the movement involves sitting back and down. Push through your heel and maintain good posture throughout the set.

Many exercisers struggle to achieve the same number the repetitions on each leg. For example, they might do 15 repetitions with the left leg and then struggle to complete 15 repetitions with the right leg because their right rectus femoris was considerably stretched while the left leg was being worked, thereby weakening the right leg and impairing its performance during the subsequent set. For this reason, I recommend always starting with the weaker leg (you should do this for any unilateral exercise), and I recommend resting about a minute between sides so you aren't impaired by stretch-related weakening.

⟨ VARIATION ⟩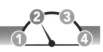

Deficit Split Squat

Once you master the traditional Bulgarian split squat, elevate the front foot on to a sturdy box or step. This allows you to sink deeper and move through even greater ranges of motion in the hip. This variation is known for inducing serious glute soreness because it provides a considerable stretch load to the muscle at the bottom of the movement. Place a pillow or folded towel under the knee of the rear leg so it doesn't crash against the floor.

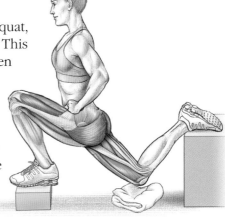

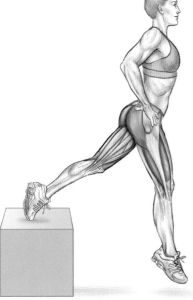

⟨ VARIATION ⟩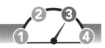

Jump Split Squat

Once you are proficient in the first two Bulgarian split-squat options, it is time to add a plyometric effect to the movement by jumping into the air. Sink all the way down, produce maximum concentric propulsion and jump as high as possible, and then absorb the landing softly.

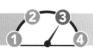

RUSSIAN LEG CURL

THIGHS

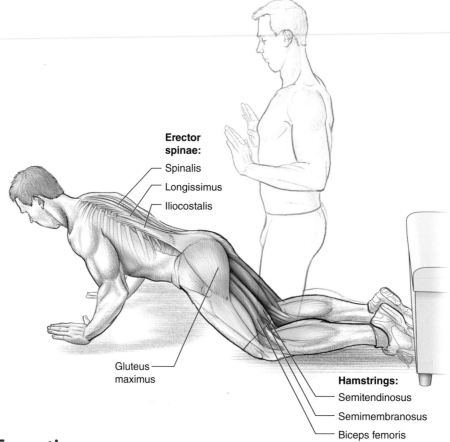

Erector spinae:
— Spinalis
— Longissimus
— Iliocostalis

Gluteus maximus

Hamstrings:
— Semitendinosus
— Semimembranosus
— Biceps femoris

Execution

1. Find a rail, beam, or stable couch to wedge your feet under. Kneel on top of a pillow or folded towel to reduce pressure on the knees.

2. With an upright trunk, lower the body under control while keeping the glutes tight, making sure not to bend forward too much at the hips or allow the pelvis to anteriorly rotate too much.

3. At the bottom of the movement, catch yourself in a push-up position and spring back to starting position, using the shoulder and arm muscles for assistance but attempting to maximize the torque on the knee joint and trying to rely on the hamstrings for movement production.

Muscles Involved

Primary: Hamstrings (biceps femoris, semitendinosus, semimembranosus)

Secondary: Erector spinae (spinalis, longissimus, iliocostalis), gluteus maximus

Exercise Notes

Think of the Russian leg curl as a bodyweight leg curl. It is an effective and challenging hamstring exercise, so much so that most beginners cannot consider performing it because of its requirement for tremendous hamstring strength. When first learning the movement you will sink very fast, which is okay. Hold proper position and attempt to lower the body slowly. Over time you'll be able to perform the movement under control.

⟨ VARIATION ⟩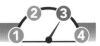

Partner-Assisted Russian Leg Curl

It helps tremendously to have a strong partner to assist with this movement. Have a partner hold the back of your ankles, bracing his or her body over your ankles and pushing down to hold you in position. As your body descends, your partner will need to brace very hard to provide the required support to secure your body so all of your energy goes into the exercise and isn't wasted trying to stabilize yourself. Lower the body slowly and push your body back to starting position while trying to use the hamstrings as much as possible. Make sure you squeeze the glutes throughout the movement to ensure that the pelvis does not tilt forward.

⟨ VARIATION ⟩

No-Hands Russian Leg Curl

The no-hands Russian leg curl is highly advanced. Most exercisers never get to this point, but with consistent training you'll be able to perform the movement all on your own. Your hamstrings will be able to produce sufficient force to reverse your body and raise it to lockout with no assistance from your arms. When you reach this point, simply place your hands behind your back. As the set progresses, put your arms at the side just in case you need to use them to prevent a face plant.

THIGHS

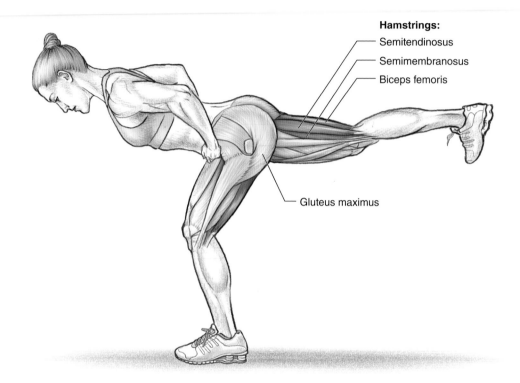

Hamstrings:
Semitendinosus
Semimembranosus
Biceps femoris

Gluteus maximus

Execution

1. Stand on one foot. Squeeze the glute of the nongrounded leg to lock it into position as it travels back.

2. Making sure the rear leg stays in line with the torso, bend over at the waist while shifting the weight back and looking down to prevent cervical hyperextension. Keep the chest up.

3. Keeping a strong low-back arch, descend until your hamstring range of motion runs out. Reverse the motion back to starting position. Perform all the repetitions on the weaker leg first and then switch and repeat with the stronger leg.

Muscles Involved

Primary: Hamstrings (biceps femoris, semitendinosus, semimembranosus)

Secondary: Erector spinae (spinalis, longissimus, iliocostalis), gluteus maximus

Exercise Notes

The single-leg Romanian deadlift uses the primary hip-hinging pattern that is required for basic lifting technique. Lifters have to learn to hinge at the hips while keeping the low back arched because this pattern is needed for many exercises. Many lifters perform this exercise incorrectly by bending the rear leg, failing to keep the rear leg in line with the rest of the body, looking up and therefore hyperextending the neck, or rounding the back. Squeeze the rear glute to lock the leg in place because there should be a straight line from the heel to the head during this movement. This serves as an excellent mobility, stability, and sensorimotor exercise because it's quite challenging to maintain proper balance.

〈 **VARIATION** 〉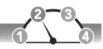

Reaching Romanian Deadlift With Knee Raise

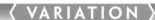

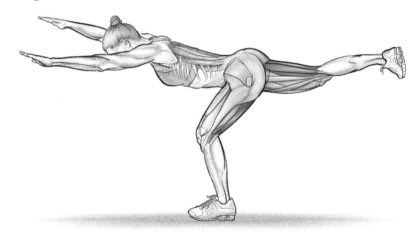

When you have mastered the single-leg Romanian deadlift, incorporate a reaching technique by flexing the shoulders to raise the arms so they're in a straight line with the rest of the body. The rear leg, torso, and arms should be roughly parallel to the ground. In addition, perform a knee lift at the top of the movement while balancing on one leg. This exercise is challenging in terms of hip and thoracic spine flexibility as well as proprioceptive control.

THIGHS

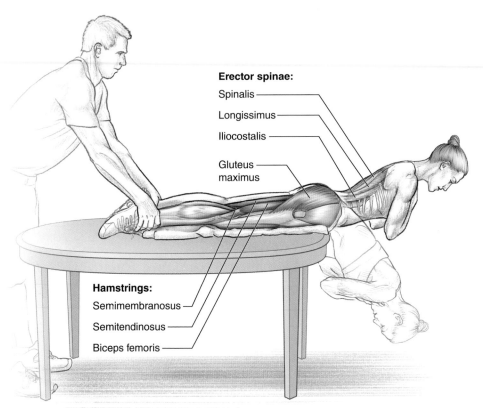

Erector spinae:
Spinalis
Longissimus
Iliocostalis

Gluteus maximus

Hamstrings:
Semimembranosus
Semitendinosus
Biceps femoris

Execution

1. With a partner holding the backs of your ankles, drape your body over the end of a couch or sturdy table so that your legs are straight and secured. Make sure the neck is in neutral position and the hands are in the mummy position (crossed in front of the body).

2. Bend at the hips and not the spine, getting a good stretch in the hamstrings.

3. Raise the torso while squeezing the glutes to lockout.

Muscles Involved

Primary: Hamstrings (biceps femoris, semitendinosus, semimembranosus), gluteus maximus

Secondary: Erector spinae (spinalis, longissimus, iliocostalis)

Exercise Notes

The partner-assisted back extension is an excellent and efficient exercise for the hamstrings, gluteals, and erector spinae. Most people perform this exercise incorrectly. Because the exercise is called a back extension, most people feel the need to flex and extend the spine to try to feel the movement in the spinal erectors as much as possible. It is more effective to make the glutes and hamstrings the prime movers by flexing and extending at the hips and keeping a rigid spine throughout the exercise. For this reason it should really be called a hip extension rather than a back extension. At the top of the motion squeeze the glutes as hard as possible and envision your glutes pulling your torso upright to erect your body. The hamstrings are critical sprinting muscles, and this exercise helps strengthen them appropriately.

⟨ **VARIATION** ⟩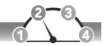

Prisoner Back Extension

Once the traditional partner-assisted back extension becomes too easy, you can increase the difficulty by placing the arms overhead and clasping the hands behind the neck in the prisoner position. This increases loading at the end of the lever and requires additional hip torque.

⟨ **VARIATION** ⟩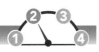

Single-Leg Back Extension

When double-leg back extensions become too easy, start performing the exercise one leg at a time. Keep the body rigid and don't allow your energy to leak through lateral or rotary motion. Feel a stretch in the hamstrings down low and squeeze the glutes hard up top. When you have mastered this variation, place the arms in the prisoner position. This movement is one of the most effective bodyweight hamstring exercises available.

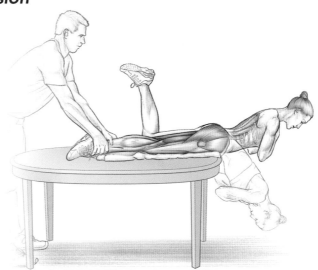

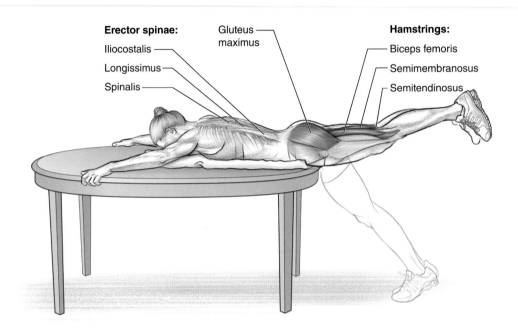

Erector spinae:
Iliocostalis
Longissimus
Spinalis

Gluteus maximus

Hamstrings:
Biceps femoris
Semimembranosus
Semitendinosus

Execution

1. Lie with your torso across a sturdy table, draping your legs over the edge and grasping the edges of the table, knees straight.

2. Keeping the torso locked into place, raise the legs, making sure to squeeze the glutes up top and prevent overextension of the low back.

3. Lower the legs to starting position, keeping the spine stable and making sure to prevent rounding the low back.

Muscles Involved

Primary: Gluteus maximus, hamstrings (biceps femoris, semitendinosus, semimembranosus)

Secondary: Erector spinae (spinalis, longissimus, iliocostalis)

Exercise Notes

The reverse hyper is an effective posterior chain exercise that works the entire back side of the body at once. Grip the edges of the table to keep your body secure and lock your spine into place. Look down to prevent hyperextending the neck. Get a big stretch in the hamstrings down low and squeeze the glutes forcefully at lockout. When done properly, the reverse hyper is an amazing lower-body and core movement that is highly beneficial to the spine.

⟨ VARIATION ⟩

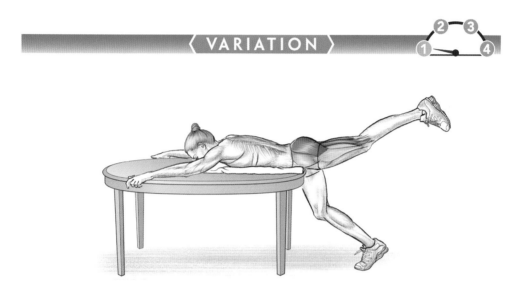

Single-Leg Reverse Hyper

For people who struggle with the double-leg reverse hyper, the single-leg reverse hyper is easier because it requires less from the spinal erectors. Focus on keeping proper body position and moving solely at the hips and not the spine. Soon you'll be able to perform double-leg reverse hypers, but make sure you master the single-leg version first.

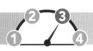

SLIDING LEG CURL

THIGHS

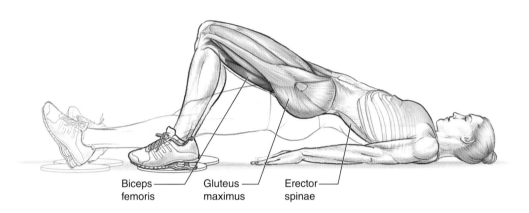

Biceps femoris   Gluteus maximus   Erector spinae

Execution

1. Lie on your back with palms down, placing your heels on two paper plates. You also may use commercially-available sliding exercise discs or, on a slick floor, two small hand towels.

2. Bridge upward in the hips while simultaneously bringing the heels toward the buttocks.

3. Keep the hips high throughout the movement. Lower the body back to starting position.

Muscles Involved

Primary: Hamstrings (biceps femoris, semitendinosus, semimembranosus)

Secondary: Erector spinae (spinalis, longissimus, iliocostalis), gluteus maximus

Exercise Notes

The sliding leg curl is an effective hamstring exercise that develops both hip extension and knee flexion strength at the same time. Most people perform this exercise incorrectly by sagging at the hips and failing to keep the hips extended throughout the set. Proper form takes advanced levels of strength and discipline because it's tempting to allow the hips to drop and simply flex and extend the knees. Squeeze the glutes to raise the hips and keep them contracted while pulling the feet toward the rear with the hamstrings. Some strong people can perform this movement one leg at a time. Not me.

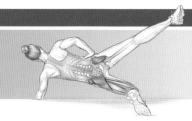

chapter 8

GLUTES

Over the past several years, I've become known as the Glute Guy. I'd be surprised if I met anyone who is equally or more interested in the glutes than I. I have conducted thousands of hours of research, including poring over scientific literature and hooking myself up to electrodes to measure the glutes' electromyography activity during exercise. More important, I've helped hundreds of clients dramatically improve the strength and shape of their glutes. This transformation is critical for men who seek an athletic appearance because strong glutes produce powerful locomotion. Along the same lines, a woman with firm, sculpted buttocks is sure to catch everyone's attention. An appealing backside continues to become more popular as evidenced by the numerous references in song lyrics and attention in the media.

GLUTEAL MUSCLES

The glutes consist of three muscles: the gluteus maximus, gluteus medius, and gluteus minimus. (See figure 7.1*b* to see the location of the glutes in relation to the back of the upper leg.) It is often said that the gluteus maximus is the strongest and most powerful muscle in the human body. As humans evolved and began walking upright on two legs, their glutes developed. Further gluteal development occurred as humans gained coordination and learned to use the glutes when sprinting, throwing, and swinging things, and now our gluteus maximus muscles are the best developed of all of the primates. Unfortunately, because of today's sedentary lifestyle, many people possess weak and underdeveloped glutes. Don't fall into that trap. Understand that the gluteus maximus is responsible for several joint actions. Concentric contractions (muscle fibers shorten) extend the hip, laterally rotate the hip, abduct the hip (move leg away from center of body), and posteriorly (toward front) tilt the pelvis. The gluteus maximus functions isometrically (with little shortening of muscle) and eccentrically (muscle lengthens during contraction) to prevent or absorb hip flexion and to produce internal hip rotation, hip adduction (brings leg toward center of body), and anterior (backward) pelvic tilt. The gluteus medius and gluteus minimus are responsible for hip abduction in addition to hip rotation, either internal or external depending on the muscle fibers and level of hip flexion.

All of the gluteal muscles possess several functional subdivisions, meaning that the various fibers within the muscles can function separately in order to carry out different actions. For example, the upper gluteus maximus fibers are highly involved in hip abduction, whereas the lower gluteus maximus fibers aren't involved in this joint action. Because of the connections with the thoracolumbar fascia, iliotibial band, and sacrotuberous ligaments, the gluteus maximus plays important roles in foot and ankle mechanics and power transfer from the upper to lower body during the gait cycle.

Not only are the glutes the powerhouse of the human body, but they're also the keystone muscles that keep everything else in line. Strong gluteals are critical for a properly functioning body. Weak glutes have been associated with myriad dysfunctional movement patterns. It is important that the knees track properly over the toes when climbing, stepping, jumping, landing, and squatting. Because the glutes contract during hip movement to prevent the knees from caving in (valgus collapse), weak glutes can lead to knee pain caused by excessive stress in the patellofemoral region if this repetitive dysfunctional pattern occurs. Furthermore, strong glutes will shift movement patterns to absorb and produce more force at the hips and less at the knee joint. For example, people with strong hips will sit back more in a squat, whereas people who are quad dominant or simply have weak hip extensors will stay more upright and bend more forward at the knees, which over time can lead to knee pain.

It is also important to keep the spine in a relatively neutral position during bending and lifting tasks, maintaining the normal, natural curvature of the lumbar spine. People with strong glutes are more apt to keep a rigid neutral spine when lifting and move mostly around the hip joint, whereas people with weak glutes are more likely to round excessively at the lower back (lumbar compensation), which over time can lead to lower back pain. Sacroiliac (SI) joint pain is often caused by weak glutes. Because the gluteus maximus pulls the ligaments taut to sufficiently close the SI joint, exercisers with weak glutes are more prone to SI joint instability during strenuous activity, which can cause pain.

Strong glutes exert a posterior pull on the pelvis to help maintain proper posture. Weak glutes can lead to what's been coined *lower-crossed syndrome*. This postural distortion is characterized by imbalanced muscle pairs, called force couples, across the lumbopelvic region. Essentially, the pull of the spinal erectors and hip flexors, which anteriorly tilt the pelvis, exceeds the pull of the glutes and abdominals, which posteriorly tilt the pelvis, causing a gradual anterior pelvic tilt over time accompanied by hyperlordosis (overarching) of the lumbar spine, thereby predisposing the body to lower back pain.

The gluteus maximus pulls rearward on the upper femur during hip extension, and people with weak glutes are likely to suffer from anterior hip pain caused by jamming the head of the femur into the front of the hip socket during hip extension. This is known as *anterior femoral glide syndrome*. Depending on the task, insufficient glute strength can require more output from the quadriceps, hip adductors, hamstrings, hip rotators, quadratus lumborum, erector spinae, and even the abdominals. This can lead to various tears in the surrounding muscles because of a phenomenon called *synergistic dominance*. For example, a pulled biceps femoris of the hamstrings or adductor magnus during sprinting could be the result of the muscle being overworked as it tries to pick up the slack for a weak gluteus maximus.

The term *gluteal amnesia* describes the status of the backsides of today's weak, poorly developed, and sedentary people whose glutes are so atrophied and uncoordinated that they fail to work properly during functional movement. This lack of functional coordination occurs for myriad reasons. Excessive sitting decreases flexibility in the hip extensors, inhibits gluteal activation, and compresses gluteal tissue, thereby shutting off its blood supply, which interferes with nutrient delivery and neural functioning. Finally, the law of use vs. disuse applies heavily to the glutes; people who use the muscles of their buttocks keep them, but folks who fail to use them will watch their glutes wither away over time.

GLUTES IN MOTION

The glutes are vital for functional movement. Walking, standing up from a chair, climbing stairs, picking up objects off the floor, and carrying objects across the room all require properly functioning posterior chain musculature. (The spinal erectors, gluteus maximus, and hamstrings make up the posterior chain.) The gluteus maximus plays a major role in most athletic activities. As an athlete matures from novice to advanced to elite status, he or she learns to derive increasing amounts of propulsive power from the hips. Propulsive power is considerably influenced by the strength of the gluteus maximus because this muscle is heavily involved in nearly all primary sporting motions including running, cutting, jumping, throwing, and striking.

The gluteus maximus contracts forcefully to extend the hips during foot strike in a sprint, during a countermovement vertical jump, while freestyle swimming or hiking a mountain, and to buck an opponent out of a full-mount position in mixed martial arts. The external rotational power of the gluteus maximus produces the twisting torque at the hips required to forcefully swing a bat in baseball or softball or racket in tennis, to throw a ball in American football or baseball, to heave a shot put, discuss, or hammer in track and field, or to throw a hook, cross, or uppercut in boxing. The abduction power of the gluteus maximus produces lateral stability during running to prevent hip sag in addition to producing lateral power when cutting from side to side during agility and change-of-direction maneuvers in sports such as American football, soccer, volleyball, basketball, hockey, and tennis.

Not only is the gluteus maximus involved in high-power and speed sports such as track and field, it also is used in high-force sports such as powerlifting and strongman. Heavy squatting, deadlifting, stone lifting, and carrying require intense gluteus maximus strength. In Olympic weightlifting, cleaning, jerking, and snatching actions require substantial gluteus maximus power to accelerate the barbell.

What's more, the gluteus maximus functions concentrically, eccentrically, and isometrically during sporting actions to produce and reduce force. It also prevents energy leaks, which maximizes movement efficiency. Sure, sporting movement requires that your muscles work in a coordinated and synergistic fashion. And yes, many muscles are important for producing power and speed, such as the quadriceps during jumping and the hamstrings during sprint running. That said, an excellent case could be made that the gluteus maximus is the most versatile and important muscle for total athleticism because of its multiple functions at the hips.

Bodyweight exercises can build the glutes very well, but it's important to first learn proper form during basic exercises before advancing to more difficult variations. Many people fail to properly activate their glutes or use movement strategies to take advantage of the strong and powerful gluteus maximus. By mastering proper activation and using excellent technical form, you will rely on the gluteus maximus for many primal movement patterns, including squatting, bending, lunging, twisting, walking, and running. It is often said that abs are made in the kitchen. I'm here to tell you that glutes are made during strength training exercise.

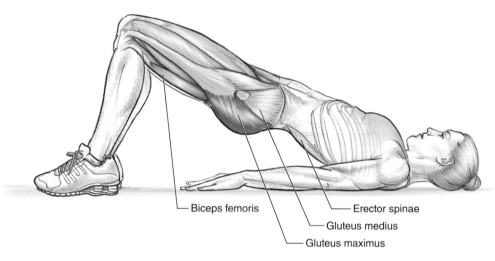

Biceps femoris — Erector spinae — Gluteus medius — Gluteus maximus

Execution

1. Lie on your back with the knees bent at 90 degrees and the palms flat on the ground.
2. Pushing through the heels, raise the hips as high as possible using the gluteal muscles. Move solely around the hip joint and keep the lower back in a neutral position.
3. Hold the bridge in the top position for a moment, then lower the hips to starting position.

Muscles Involved

Primary: Gluteus maximus

Secondary: Hamstrings (biceps femoris, semitendinosus, semimembranosus), erector spinae (spinalis, longissimus, iliocostalis), adductor magnus, adductor longus, adductor brevis, gluteus medius, gluteus minimus

Exercise Notes

The glute bridge is the fundamental bent-leg hip extension movement on which all bridging motions are built. The goal is to feel the glutes lifting the hips and not the hamstrings or spinal erectors. Avoid hyperextending the lumbar spine or anteriorly tilting the pelvis. Bending the knees shortens the hamstring muscle, reducing its contribution to the movement and putting more emphasis on the gluteus maximus. Many people initially feel their hamstrings cramp during bridging movements because their hamstrings aren't accustomed to bent-leg hip extension motions. This quickly dissipates as the glutes learn to take on a primary hip extension role and the hamstrings serve a secondary role. Strong, activated glutes prevent forward pelvic tilting and low-back overarching, which is critical for optimal performance during this exercise.

⟨ VARIATION ⟩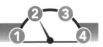

Glute March

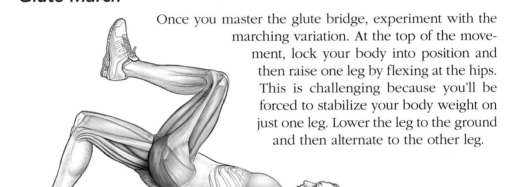

Once you master the glute bridge, experiment with the marching variation. At the top of the movement, lock your body into position and then raise one leg by flexing at the hips. This is challenging because you'll be forced to stabilize your body weight on just one leg. Lower the leg to the ground and then alternate to the other leg.

⟨ VARIATION ⟩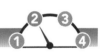

Single-Leg Glute Bridge

After you've become proficient at the glute march, move on to the single-leg glute bridge. Simply keep one leg bent 90 degrees at the hip and knee and perform the bridging movement on one leg. After completing all the repetitions, repeat with the other leg.

SHOULDER-ELEVATED HIP THRUST

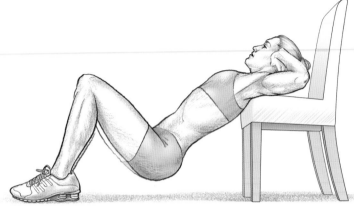

Starting position.

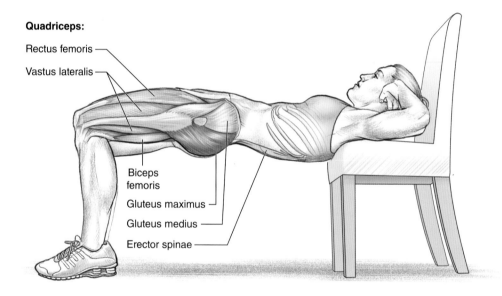

Quadriceps:

Rectus femoris

Vastus lateralis

Biceps femoris

Gluteus maximus

Gluteus medius

Erector spinae

Execution

1. Facing upward, place your upper back on top of a couch, sturdy chair, or weight bench with your feet flat on the ground.

2. Place the hands on the ears and extend the hips by squeezing the glutes. Push through the heels and keep the lower back in a neutral position.

3. Rise as high as possible through the hips and then lower your hips to starting position.

Muscles Involved

Primary: Gluteus maximus

Secondary: Hamstrings (biceps femoris, semitendinosus, semimembranosus), erector spinae (spinalis, longissimus, iliocostalis), adductor magnus, adductor longus, adductor brevis, gluteus medius, gluteus minimus, quadriceps (rectus femoris, vastus lateralis, vastus medialis, vastus intermedius)

Exercise Notes

The shoulder-elevated hip thrust improves on the basic hip thrust by increasing the demands at the hip and knee joints. This variation is more difficult for the quadriceps and moves the hips through a greater range of motion than the floor version. The most difficult portion of the movement is the top, which is characterized by a neutral or slightly hyperextended hip position. It is important to be strong in this range of motion because it is used when running. Comparatively, this range of hip motion is not strengthened during the squat exercises because there are no hip extension torque requirements at the hip in neutral position when standing. For this reason, the squat and hip thrust exercises complement each other well.

⟨ VARIATION ⟩

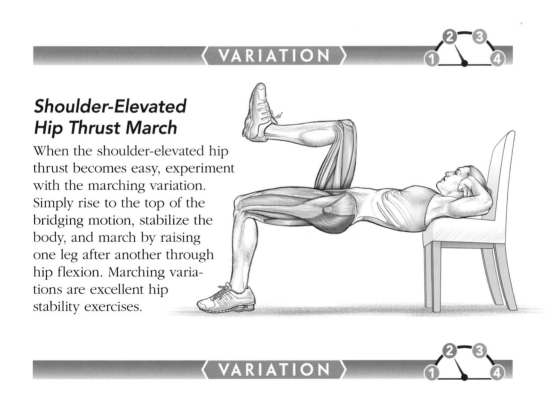

Shoulder-Elevated Hip Thrust March

When the shoulder-elevated hip thrust becomes easy, experiment with the marching variation. Simply rise to the top of the bridging motion, stabilize the body, and march by raising one leg after another through hip flexion. Marching variations are excellent hip stability exercises.

⟨ VARIATION ⟩

Single-Leg Hip Thrust

Once the marching variation is no longer challenging, perform the single-leg hip thrust. This is an advanced variation that requires considerable hip extension strength and rotary stability in the lumbopelvic region. Rise up all the way; many exercisers skimp on their range of motion when this movement gets difficult.

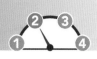

SHOULDER-AND-FEET-ELEVATED HIP THRUST

GLUTES

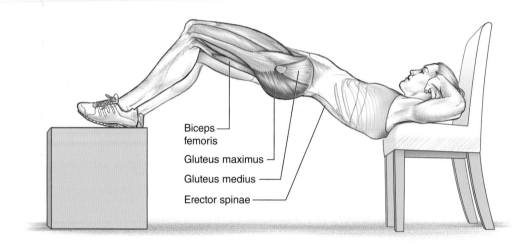

Biceps femoris

Gluteus maximus

Gluteus medius

Erector spinae

Execution

1. Facing upward, place your upper back on a couch, sturdy chair, or weight bench and your feet on a small table, stool, or chair. The two surfaces should be roughly the same height.

2. Extend the hips by squeezing the glutes. Push through the heels and keep the lower back neutral.

3. Rise as high as possible through the hips and then lower the hips to starting position.

Muscles Involved

Primary: Gluteus maximus

Secondary: Hamstrings (biceps femoris, semitendinosus, semimembranosus), erector spinae (spinalis, longissimus, iliocostalis), adductor magnus, adductor longus, adductor brevis, gluteus medius, gluteus minimus

Exercise Notes

The shoulder-and-feet-elevated hip thrust is the most challenging bridging variation because it moves the hips through the greatest range of motion and considerably increases the demands on the hamstrings. The double-leg version is still challenging for many intermediate-level exercisers, although more advanced exercisers will require single-leg variations to sufficiently challenge their hip extensors. The reason the hamstrings work so much harder in this variation is because the hips drop lower than the feet, thereby requiring the hamstrings to produce a knee flexion torque as well as a hip extension torque. For this reason, this exercise works the hamstrings through both of its roles—hip extension and knee flexion.

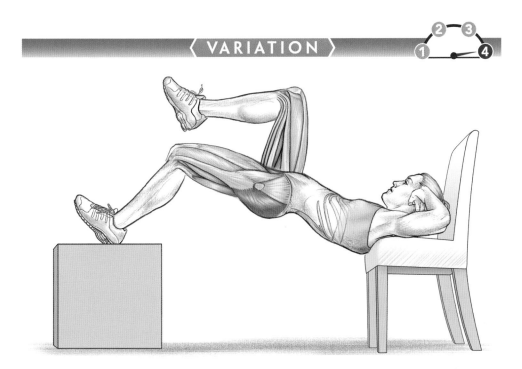

‹ VARIATION ›

Single-Leg Shoulder-and-Feet-Elevated Hip Thrust

Once you reach proficiency in the double-leg shoulder-and-feet-elevated hip thrust, you can try the single-leg version. Many people foolishly rush into this variation before they're ready for it. The single-leg shoulder-and-feet-elevated hip thrust is likely the most challenging bodyweight exercise for the hips because it requires tremendous gluteal strength and stability. Frankly, most beginners and even most intermediate exercisers don't possess this. Take your time moving up through the exercise progressions so by the time you start performing the single-leg shoulder-and-feet-elevated hip thrust you can perform it correctly. This means moving the hips through a controlled and full range of motion while preventing lateral and rotational energy leaks. Pause briefly at the top of each repetition to ensure proper performance.

GLUTES

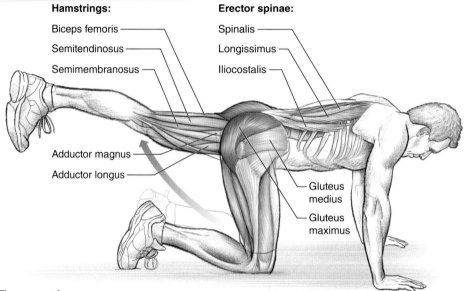

Hamstrings:
Biceps femoris
Semitendinosus
Semimembranosus

Adductor magnus
Adductor longus

Erector spinae:
Spinalis
Longissimus
Iliocostalis

Gluteus medius

Gluteus maximus

Execution

1. Start on all fours (quadruped position) with the head, neck, and spine in neutral position, the hands under the shoulders and the knees under the hips. No flexion, extension, lateral flexion, or rotation in the neck and spine.

2. Kick one leg to the rear until you reach full extension.

3. Return to starting position. Complete all repetitions on one leg before switching legs.

Muscles Involved

Primary: Gluteus maximus

Secondary: Hamstrings (biceps femoris, semitendinosus, semimembranosus), erector spinae (spinalis, longissimus, iliocostalis), adductor magnus, adductor longus, adductor brevis, gluteus medius, gluteus minimus, multifidus

Exercise Notes

The donkey kick is a basic hip extension exercise that trains your ability to keep the spine and pelvis in neutral while the hips move through their full range of motion. Many beginners struggle with these movements because they're used to compensating with their erector spinae by anteriorly tilting the pelvis and hyperextending the lumbar spine. This creates the illusion of full hip extension, but on closer inspection full hip extension hasn't been reached. It is important to learn how to extend at the hips while keeping the spine and pelvis relatively neutral.

‹ VARIATION ›

Bent-Leg Donkey Kick

The bent-leg donkey kick, in which the knee is bent to 90 degrees while the leg is lifted, shortens the hamstrings and reduces the participation of the hamstrings in the movement. Because the hamstrings are weakened, the stronger glutes will pick up the slack, which makes this movement a more targeted glute exercise because it requires less hamstring and spinal erector torque while keeping the tension on the glutes. Squeeze the glutes at the top of the movement and keep the spine straight as the hip rises.

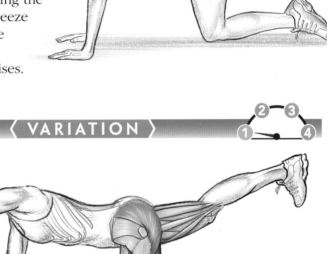

‹ VARIATION ›

Bird Dog

The bird dog exercise builds on the donkey kick by adding a diagonal upper-body movement pattern to complement the lower-body movement and allow for proper transfer through the core. During this movement alternate between extension patterns of diagonal pairs—left arm combined with right leg and right arm combined with left leg. The diagonal movement patterns call on the spinal stabilizers to resist rotational movement, which makes for an effective core-stability exercise.

GLUTES

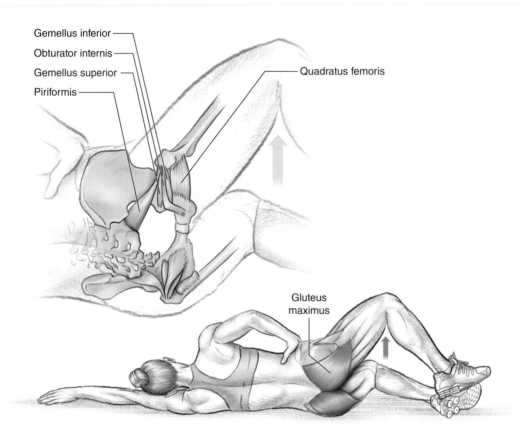

SIDE-LYING CLAM

Gemellus inferior
Obturator internis
Gemellus superior
Piriformis

Quadratus femoris

Gluteus maximus

Execution

1. Start in a side-lying position with the hips bent at about 135 degrees and the knees bent at about 90 degrees. The neck rests on the arm on the ground. The other arm is braced on top of the hip.

2. With the heels touching each other, rotate the top hip up. Be sure to move at the hips. Don't lean to one side or move at the spine. The heels stay together for the entire set.

3. Return to starting position. Complete the desired number of repetitions and repeat on the other side.

Muscles Involved

Primary: Gluteus maximus

Secondary: Deep-hip external rotators (piriformis, gemellus superior, obturator internus, gemellus inferior, obturator externus, quadratus femoris)

Exercise Notes

The side-lying clam is a surprisingly effective exercise and is a favorite warm-up movement of many of my female clients because they like to feel the burn in their glutes. When performed correctly the movement create a good burn in both the gluteus maximus and the external hip rotators. Many people perform the exercise inefficiently by losing contact between the heels or leaning to the rear. This is a short-range movement that will strengthen external hip rotation, a critical joint action in sports.

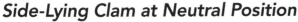

⟨ VARIATION ⟩

Side-Lying Clam at Neutral Position

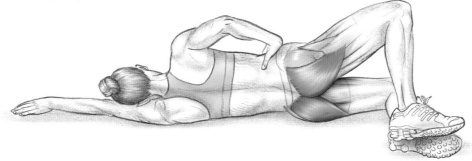

The side-lying clam can also be performed in a hips-neutral manner by keeping a rather straight line from the shoulders to the knees. Keep the heels in contact with each other through the duration of the set and avoid leaning or twisting at the spine.

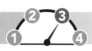
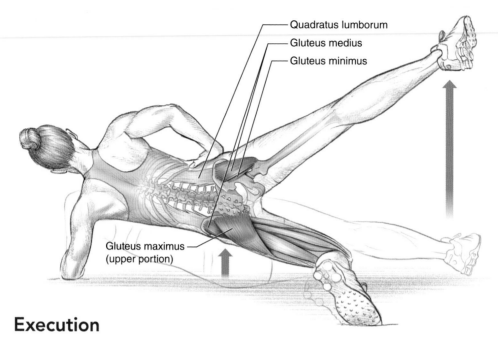

Quadratus lumborum
Gluteus medius
Gluteus minimus
Gluteus maximus (upper portion)

GLUTES

Execution

1. From a side-lying position, lift up onto the lower elbow and place the hand of the other arm on the hip.

2. Making sure that the body is in a straight line from the shoulders to the knees, raise the body by simultaneously abducting the bottom and the top hips.

3. Lower yourself to starting position. Complete the desired number of repetitions and repeat on the other side.

Muscles Involved

Primary: Gluteus medius, gluteus minimus, upper gluteus maximus

Secondary: Internal oblique, external oblique, quadratus lumborum

Exercise Notes

The side-lying hip raise is an advanced movement that strengthens the upper glutes and core musculature. Keep a neutral hip position and avoid flexing forward at the hips. The bottom knee will always be bent, but the top knee can be bent (easier version) or straight (more difficult version), depending on the desired level of difficulty. Control the body through a full range of motion and avoid jerky movements. This exercise strengthens hip abduction, which is a critical joint action in sports.

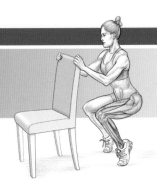

chapter 9

CALVES

The calves are a unique muscle group. Many people find that no matter what they do, they struggle to grow their calves, whereas certain lucky people don't even have to train them directly to achieve impressive lower-leg development. A substantial genetic component affects calf aesthetics, and it's difficult to override your genetic blueprint. Favorable genetics for calf development provide long muscle bellies, short Achilles tendons, and favourable fast-twitch to slow-twitch fiber ratios. However, many people have overcome their limits and developed impressive calves through hard work and consistency. For example, Arnold Schwarzenegger used to hide his calves when he was photographed but was eventually able to turn his poor calf development into a strong point by working the muscles relentlessly with an aggressive combination of volume, intensity, and frequency.

If you're one of the lucky ones who don't have to perform direct calf work to sport muscular calves, then chances are you take this genetic gift for granted. But if you have toothpicks for lower limbs, then you'd probably go to great lengths to achieve muscular symmetry in this area of the body. It's important to possess at the bare minimum a basic level of strength and development in the lower limbs.

If you think of walking as a short-range bodyweight calf raise, then you'll realize how acclimated the calves are to low-intensity training. A typical American takes an average of 7,000 steps per day (compared to 18,000 steps per day in the Amish population). To get the calves to grow, you need to use strategies that place maximum tension on the calf muscles because they're already quite accustomed to activities of lower intensity.

CALF MUSCLES

When people speak of the calves, they typically refer to the gastrocnemius and soleus muscles (figure 9.1). These two muscles and the plantaris muscle, a muscle that is only 2 to 4 inches (5-10 cm) long and is absent in about 10 percent of the population, share a common tendon, the Achilles tendon. The gastrocnemius has two distinct heads: the lateral head and the medial head. The soleus lies under the gastrocnemius and is a monoarticular muscle that crosses only the ankle joint, so it is not mechanically affected by the knee angle. The same cannot be said of the gastrocnemius, which is a biarticular muscle that crosses the ankle and knee joints and is therefore shortened and inhibited when the knee is bent. For this reason, bent-knee exercises that use plantar flexion (bends foot downward) such as the seated calf raise exercise targets the soleus muscle and not the gastrocnemius muscle.

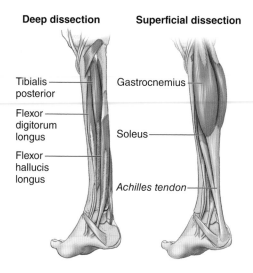

Deep dissection

Tibialis posterior

Flexor digitorum longus

Flexor hallucis longus

Superficial dissection

Gastrocnemius

Soleus

Achilles tendon

a

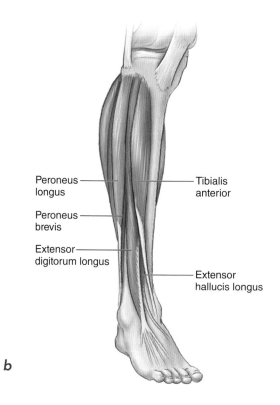

Peroneus longus

Peroneus brevis

Extensor digitorum longus

Tibialis anterior

Extensor hallucis longus

b

Figure 9.1 Lower leg muscles: *(a)* back, including both deep and superficial dissection, and *(b)* front.

Although the soleus and gastrocnemius both serve as plantarflexors (they elevate the heel when standing), only the gastrocnemius can produce mild knee flexion, especially when the knee is more extended. Many other lower leg muscles assist in plantarflexion, including the plantaris, peroneus longus, peroneus brevis, flexor hallucis longus, flexor digitorum longus, and tibialis posterior.

Compared to the gastrocnemius, the soleus generally has a much greater percentage of slow-twitch fibers and thus has been shown to initiate slow contractions. The gastrocnemius tends to initiate faster contractions. It is possible to target the lateral or medial head of the gastrocnemius by varying foot position. An externally rotated position (feet pointed out) activates the more medial (toward center of the body) gastrocnemius, whereas an internally rotated position (feet pointed in) activates the more lateral (toward the outside of the body) gastrocnemius.

CALF ACTIONS

The calf muscles are used during low-level activity such as standing and walking, and they provide a considerable amount of stability for balance. In sports, the calf muscles are highly activated when running, jumping, sprinting, and cutting from side to side. The soleus has been shown to be more important for vertical jumping than the gastrocnemius. The gastrocnemius has been shown to be highly activated during the propulsive phase of ground contact in sprinting. Therefore, you should strengthen both muscles. For sport purposes, it is important to not only possess strength in the lower leg musculature, but also power and stability. Plyometric activities, which repeatedly and rapidly contract and stretch the muscles, will help increase these qualities.

ELEVATED CALF RAISE

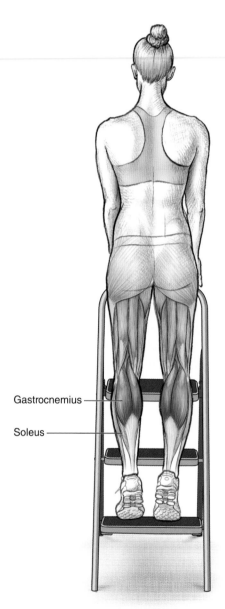

Gastrocnemius

Soleus

Execution

1. Begin with the toes on a platform or step and the body upright.

2. While grasping something for balance, lower the body and feel a good stretch in the calves.

3. Raise the body as high as possible on the toes, holding the top position for a 1-second count. Repeat until the desired number of repetitions is completed.

Muscles Involved

Primary: Gastrocnemius

Secondary: Soleus

Exercise Notes

The elevated calf raise is an excellent exercise and can be done using high repetitions. Many people skimp on their range of motion with this movement. Sink deep and rise all the way up when you perform this exercise. Sometimes you can perform faster repetitions that are more bouncy, while other times you can perform the repetitions under strict control, holding the top position for extended times and lowering the body very slowly for an accentuated eccentric component.

⟨ VARIATION ⟩

Single-Leg Elevated Calf Raise

Once the double-leg elevated calf raise becomes easy, move to the single-leg variation. Make sure you sink into this movement and load up the working leg to its full potential. Remember to pause for a second at the top of the repetition. I still struggle to achieve 20 repetitions of this movement.

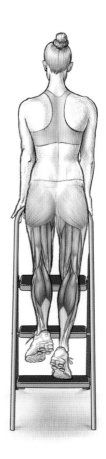

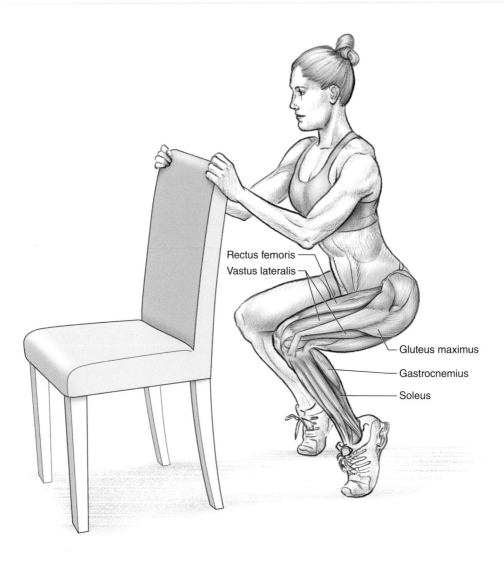

SQUAT CALF RAISE

Rectus femoris
Vastus lateralis

Gluteus maximus

Gastrocnemius

Soleus

Execution

1. Begin with your weight on your toes and sink into a parallel squat position so the knees are bent to about 90 degrees.

2. While grasping something for balance and holding the hip and knee position steady, lower the body at the ankle and feel a good stretch at the ankle joint.

3. Raise the body as high as possible onto the toes, holding the top position for a 1-second count. Repeat until the desired number of repetitions is completed.

Muscles Involved

Primary: Soleus

Secondary: Gastrocnemius, quadriceps (rectus femoris, vastus lateralis, vastus medialis, vastus intermedius), gluteus maximus

Exercise Notes

The squat calf raise takes the gastrocnemius muscle out of the movement and targets the soleus for muscle activation. This movement is a little tricky, so focus on proper form. Keep your hip and knee angles in a static position while moving solely at the ankle joint. This requires getting used to because you'll initially want to squat up and down by extending the hips and knees. Keep the hips and knees in place and raise the body through plantar flexion only. The quadriceps and glutes get a good isometric workout during this exercise.

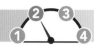
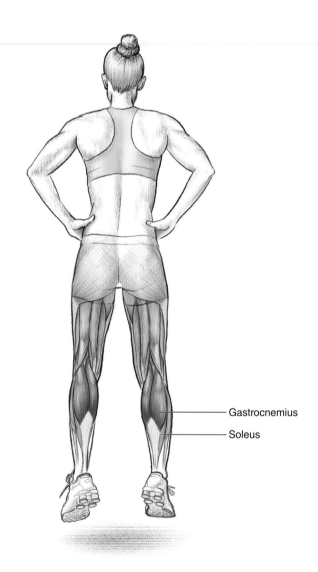

Gastrocnemius

Soleus

Execution

1. Stand with the hands at the sides or on the hips and feet shoulder-width apart.
2. Hop straight up and down, keeping the knees and hips relatively straight while trying to rely solely on the calf muscles to propel the body up.
3. Repeat until the desired amount of time has passed or number of repetitions is reached.

Muscles Involved

Primary: Gastrocnemius

Secondary: Soleus

Exercise Notes

The stiff-leg ankle hop is a good plyometric exercise for the calf musculature. Get in a rhythm and act like a pogo stick, using the calves to spring up and down. Don't bend too much at the knees and hips, which brings in the quadriceps and glutes. Although the knees will bend slightly, stay upright and focus on using the calves for movement.

⟨ VARIATION ⟩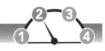

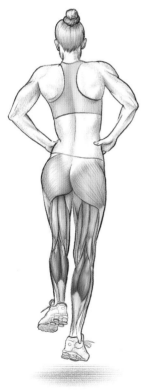

Single-Leg Ankle Hop

Once double-leg hopping becomes easy, start performing the movement one leg at a time. This is a much more demanding task and requires considerably more calf muscle strength and power. If you find yourself appearing sloppy and wasting energy during this movement, return to the double-leg version until you're ready to progress to single-leg hopping.

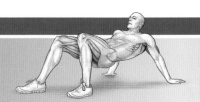

chapter 10

WHOLE BODY

Believe it or not, studies show that aerobic exercise does not provide much of an advantage to weight loss over diet alone. If weight loss is the sole objective, tightening up your diet is the quickest route to success. However, the goal of many people is to optimize body composition, or the ratio of muscle to fat. For this reason, you must take into consideration both dietary and training practices. Maintaining muscle mass while shedding excess body fat is the key to achieving a lean, defined physique.

To increase muscle size and improve muscle shape, progressive overload through strength training is imperative. Progressive overload simply means that you continuously challenge your body to do more over time, thereby forcing the muscles to adapt by becoming stronger and larger. When using your body weight for resistance, progressive overload can come in the form of advancing to more challenging exercises or exercise variations or simply performing more repetitions. This ensures that you build or maintain your muscle mass over time while simultaneously losing body fat.

Dietary practices are important as well, and adequate consumption of the proper ratio and quantities of protein, carbohydrate, and dietary fat will help maximize your muscularity and leanness. Most people find that if they center most of their meals on lean meats, fish, and vegetables, with proper amounts of fruit, dairy, and nuts added to the equation, they can't go wrong. Avoid consuming too much sugar and trans-fatty acids, and keep your overall caloric intake in check. Many people consume too much carbohydrate and could benefit from decreasing carbohydrate (especially sugar) intake while slightly increasing protein and healthy fat intake.

METABOLIC TRAINING

While diet and strength are critical in achieving your ideal physique, you should add metabolic training, another valuable factor, to the mix. Metabolic training increases the efficiency of the body's three energy systems: the creatine phosphate system, the glycolytic system, and the aerobic system. Every time you exercise you use various proportions of all three systems. However, the type of exercise employed determines which energy system is used predominantly. For example, Olympic weightlifting relies mostly on the creatine phosphate system, whereas jogging relies mostly on the aerobic system. In general, the creatine phosphate system is used to the highest degree when performing all-out efforts lasting up to 10 seconds. At this point, energy demands shift more toward the glycolytic system. And after a few minutes, sustained energy comes mostly from the aerobic system. Again, all three energy systems contribute toward the total energy pool during any form of exercise, but specific types of training are ideal for targeting one system or another.

High-Intensity Interval Training (HIIT)

Many methods exist under the metabolic training umbrella. Long slow cardio is one method that focuses on the aerobic system. Whereas short sprints with long rest periods between bouts target the creatine phosphate system. Many systems do a great job of targeting all three systems with predominance toward the glycolytic system, which is important for maximal fat loss. One such method involves high-intensity interval training (HIIT). HIIT comes in many forms, including interval sprint running, interval cycling, and interval swimming. HIIT typically alternates between periods of high intensity ranging from 10 to 40 seconds and periods of low intensity ranging from 30 to 120 seconds. For example, a session could involve 10 bouts of 30 seconds of high-intensity work sandwiched between 60 seconds of low-intensity work. Ultimately, the length of each component is your choice.

One study of the effects of HIIT showed that subjects' metabolic rates were elevated 21 percent 24 hours after and 19 percent 48 hours after an intense HIIT session. Another study showed that when taking into account the calories burned aerobically during exercise in addition to the calories burned aerobically after exercise (excess postexercise oxygen consumption, or EPOC) and the anaerobic calories burned from exercise, an aerobic exercise challenge lasting three and a half minutes burned 39 calories compared to 65 calories for three workequivalent 15-second sprints. What makes the results exceptionally appealing is the fact that HIIT burned more calories despite the fact that the total work time was roughly one-fourth that of the slower cardio session (45 seconds compared to 210 seconds).

Metabolic Resistance Training (MRT)

Resistance training is also an effective form of metabolic training, and there are ways to shift your resistance training to maximize fat loss at the expense of building a bit less muscle. This form of training is called metabolic resistance training (MRT) and is similar to HIIT training in that it creates a considerable afterburn by raising levels of EPOC.

You should take into account a few tricks of the trade in order to optimize the efficiency of MRT:

1. Perform circuits that use compound exercises, or exercises that work a lot of muscles at the same time.
2. Alternate between lower- and upper-body exercises. This allows your heart to constantly shuttle blood throughout the body while allowing individual muscles to rest so they can recharge between bouts.

3. Incorporate whole-body exercises because they're great for elevating the heart rate. I'll elaborate on this in the next paragraph.

4. During your sets, keep a fast pace during the concentric (muscles shorten during contraction) portion of your repetitions but carefully control the eccentric (muscles lengthen during contraction) component of the repetition. Both have been shown to be costlier from a metabolic perspective.

5. Use short rest periods between sets and exercises.

View metabolic training as targeting energy systems, not muscles. MRT workouts are not intended to optimize strength or muscle size, but rather to burn calories and elevate metabolism. When combining strength sessions with MRT sessions in the same week, you increase the potential of interfering with muscle recovery. Don't be foolish during MRT and push a certain muscle group too hard or you might experience a subpar strength workout later in the week and risk losing strength and muscularity over time.

WHOLE-BODY EXERCISES

I've discussed lower-body, upper-body, and core exercises in previous chapters. During whole-body exercises, the upper body, core, and lower body all work statically or dynamically throughout the set. For example, during the mountain climber exercise, the pressing muscles of the upper body and scapular stabilizers contract isometrically to keep the torso in position while the core and lower-body muscles contract dynamically to alternate between hip flexion and hip extension. Although this exercise isn't very challenging for any particular muscle, it is extremely challenging from a metabolic standpoint because a vast proportion of the body's musculature is working all at once. Whole-body exercises are a valuable tool that can help take your body composition to the next level.

As you gain physical fitness, your workouts will become increasingly more productive, allowing you to expend a greater amount of energy during training. This is why many athletes have trouble keeping on weight. Not only do they expend a large number of calories while exercising, they also expend considerable energy when they're resting as their bodies attempt to restore equilibrium following the metabolic disturbances created by their demanding workouts. While it's not critical or even ideal for you to be in the gym all day long or to engage in HIIT or MRT every day, a couple of brief, properly conducted HIIT or MRT sessions per week can help you take your physique to the next level. Next I will list some of the most effective whole-body exercises, and in the next chapter I will show you how to program these exercises into your arsenal.

JUMPING JACK

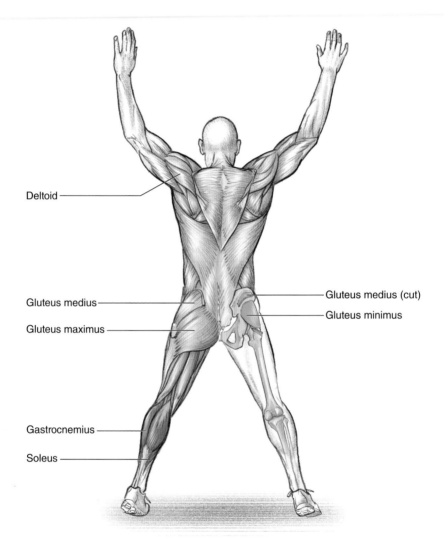

Deltoid

Gluteus medius

Gluteus maximus

Gluteus medius (cut)

Gluteus minimus

Gastrocnemius

Soleus

Execution

1. Stand with the arms to the sides and feet about hip-width apart.

2. Jump up while spreading the legs apart and raising the arms to the sides until they reach overhead.

3. Land and then spring back to starting position, bringing the legs back together and lowering the arms.

Muscles Involved

Primary: Quadriceps (rectus femoris, vastus lateralis, vastus medialis, vastus intermedius), gastrocnemius, soleus

Secondary: Deltoids, gluteus maximus, gluteus medius, gluteus minimus

Exercise Notes

The jumping jack is a classic calisthenic performed in physical education curriculum around the world. It effectively raises the metabolic rate while warming up the shoulder and hip joints. The goal is not to jump as high as possible during the jumping jack exercise but to move rhythmically and absorb the landing softly.

⟨ **VARIATION** ⟩

Transverse-Arm Jumping Jack

An alternative to the standard jumping jack is the transverse-arm jumping jack. This variation provides a better stretch for the pectorals and rear deltoids. Simply cross the arms in front of the torso as you jump up and down.

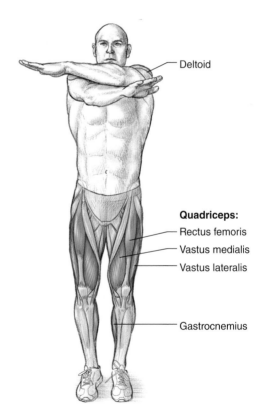

Deltoid

Quadriceps:
Rectus femoris
Vastus medialis
Vastus lateralis

Gastrocnemius

WHOLE BODY

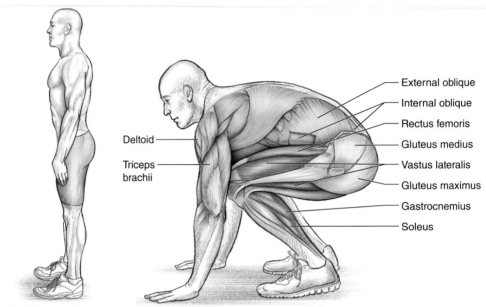

Starting position.

External oblique
Internal oblique
Rectus femoris
Gluteus medius
Vastus lateralis
Gluteus maximus
Gastrocnemius
Soleus

Deltoid
Triceps brachii

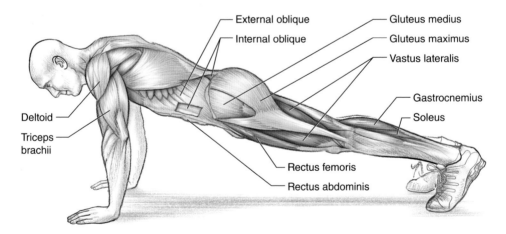

External oblique
Internal oblique
Gluteus medius
Gluteus maximus
Vastus lateralis
Gastrocnemius
Soleus
Deltoid
Triceps brachii
Rectus femoris
Rectus abdominis

Execution

1. From a standing position, squat and place your palms on the floor.
2. Kick the feet back and land in a push-up position.
3. Kick the feet forward under the hips and land in a squat position then stand up.

Muscles Involved

Primary: Quadriceps (rectus femoris, vastus lateralis, vastus medialis, vastus intermedius), gastrocnemius, soleus

Secondary: Pectoralis major, triceps brachii, rectus abdominis, internal oblique, external oblique, gluteus maximus, gluteus medius, gluteus minimus, deltoids

Exercise Notes

The burpee is a brutal conditioning exercise that will cause the heart rate to skyrocket. Although it doesn't appear to be challenging, make no mistake about it, it's grueling. Use proper form and attempt to spare the spine by avoiding excessive lumbar flexion in the bottom squat position and lumbar hyperextension in the push-up position.

⟨VARIATION⟩

Burpee With Push-Up, Jump, and Reach

If you're in good physical shape and you'd like a more advanced type of burpee, add a push-up, jump, and reach. This makes the burpee one of the most challenging conditioning exercises. From a standing position, drop into a squat, kick the feet into a push-up position, perform a push-up, kick the feet forward and land in a squat, and then jump as high as possible while reaching to the sky.

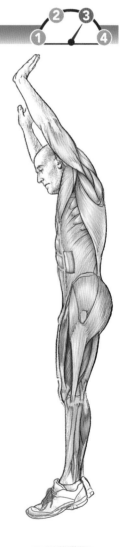

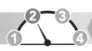

WHOLE BODY

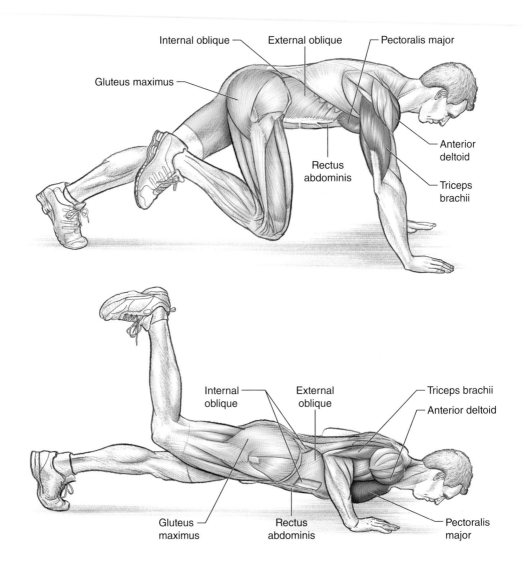

Internal oblique

External oblique

Pectoralis major

Gluteus maximus

Rectus abdominis

Anterior deltoid

Triceps brachii

Internal oblique

External oblique

Triceps brachii

Anterior deltoid

Gluteus maximus

Rectus abdominis

Pectoralis major

Execution

1. Get into the top of a push-up position. Keep the head and neck in neutral position and one leg flexed forward with the knee bent so you're maintaining three points of contact.

2. As you lower the body toward the floor, simultaneously extend the hip of the free leg while keeping the knee bent the entire time. The hip will reach peak extension at the same time the torso reaches its lowest position.

3. Rise by pressing the torso up with the pectorals, deltoids, and triceps while reversing the hip back into flexion. Complete the desired number of repetitions and repeat with the other leg.

Muscles Involved

Primary: Pectoralis major, anterior deltoid, triceps brachii

Secondary: Gluteus maximus, rectus abdominis, external oblique, internal oblique

Exercise Notes

The push-up with hip extension requires considerable coordination and muscle control. Maintain proper spinal posture throughout the set, avoiding lumbar flexion up top as one hip flexes forward and also avoiding lumbar extension down low as one hip extends back. Eventually the movement will feel comfortable as you develop the proper rhythm. This variation places additional stability demands on the spine as you to control the rotational movement caused by having only three points of support while the free leg flexes and extends.

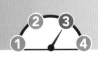

TOWEL ROW ISOHOLD
WITH GLUTE MARCH

WHOLE BODY

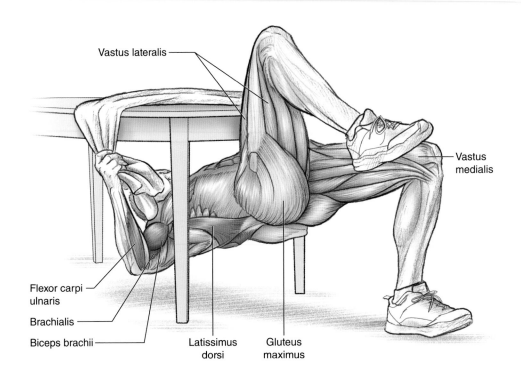

Vastus lateralis

Vastus medialis

Flexor carpi ulnaris

Brachialis

Biceps brachii

Latissimus dorsi

Gluteus maximus

Execution

1. Drape a towel over a sturdy table or weight bench that is about waist height. With the feet on the ground and the knees bent, grasp the ends of the towel and row the body up.

2. Holding the body in an isometric rowing position, lift one leg off the ground by flexing at the hip and then straightening the leg.

3. Raise the leg all the way and then lower it back down. Alternate to the other leg in a marching fashion.

Muscles Involved

Primary: Latissimus dorsi, mid trapezius, rhomboids, brachialis, biceps brachii, forearm muscles such as the flexor carpi radialis, palmaris longus, and flexor carpi ulnaris

Secondary: Erector spinae (spinalis, longissimus, iliocostalis), gluteus maximus, hip flexors (iliacus, psoas), quadriceps (rectus femoris, vastus lateralis, vastus medialis, vastus intermedius)

Exercise Notes

The towel row isohold with glute march might appear to be a simple movement, but multiple muscle groups are at work during this exercise. This creates a strong metabolic demand on the body. Keep the hips tall and maintain full hip extension throughout the set. Keep the head and neck in neutral position and keep the chest tall with the hands at the sides of the body. This exercise does an excellent job of working the entire posterior chain at once.

SIT-UP TO STAND WITH JUMP AND REACH

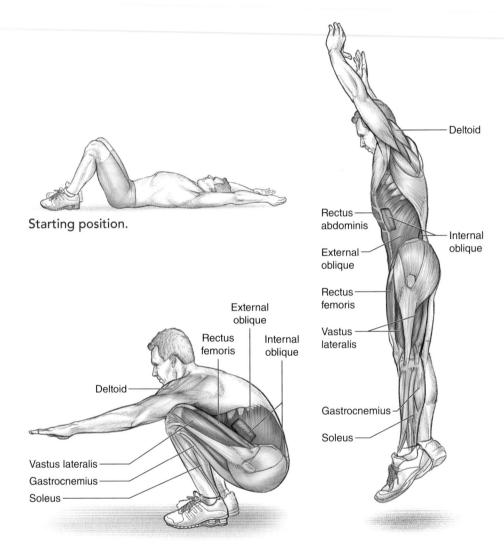

Starting position.

Deltoid

Rectus abdominis

External oblique

Internal oblique

Rectus femoris

Vastus lateralis

Gastrocnemius

Soleus

External oblique

Rectus femoris

Internal oblique

Deltoid

Vastus lateralis

Gastrocnemius

Soleus

Execution

1. Lie on your back with your arms overhead, knees bent, and feet flat on the ground. If you wish, tuck a small pillow under your buttocks. Swing the arms forward while performing an explosive sit-up maneuver.

2. Propel your body forcefully so that you're able to transition to a deep squat. Then arch the back and jump into the air while reaching the arms overhead.

3. Absorb the landing softly, squat, and gently roll the body back to starting position. Repeat for the desired number of repetitions.

Muscles Involved

Primary: Rectus abdominis, external oblique, internal oblique, quadriceps (rectus femoris, vastus lateralis, vastus medialis, vastus intermedius)

Secondary: Gastrocnemius, soleus, deltoids

Exercise Notes

The sit-up to stand with jump and reach is a highly challenging movement, especially for people with bigger torsos and less developed legs. Position a pillow under your buttocks, which will help you gently absorb the transition from the squat to sitting and back to the starting position. Jump straight up and down and avoid shifting so that your buttocks is always positioned properly in front of the pillow. Avoid moving too much in the lumbar spine and make sure your hips and upper back move the most. This will not be possible for people with limited hip flexion or limited ankle dorsiflexion, so if you find that this exercise aggravates the lower back, avoid it altogether. For people with suitable flexibility and sound levels of fitness, this exercise should not pose a problem. Keep the chest tall before jumping and absorb the shock of the landing smoothly.

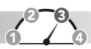
WHOLE BODY

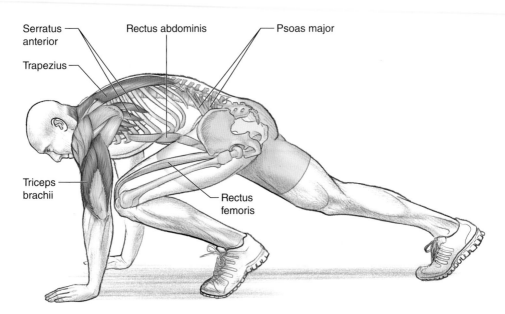

Serratus anterior — Rectus abdominis — Psoas major

Trapezius —

Triceps brachii —

Rectus femoris

Execution

1. From a standing position, bend over and place your palms on the floor.
2. Sink the hips down and straighten out one leg behind the body.
3. Alternate between jumping one leg forward by flexing the hip and kicking the other leg back by extending the hip in a climbing maneuver.

Muscles Involved

Primary: Triceps brachii, serratus anterior, trapezius

Secondary: Rectus abdominis, hip flexors (iliacus, psoas, rectus femoris)

Exercise Notes

The mountain climber is another brutal conditioning exercise. It might appear easy on the surface, but performing the mountain climber for an extended period of time is challenging. Keep the head and neck in a neutral position and move mostly at the hips and not too much at the lumbar spine. Many people cheat on this movement to make it easier by hiking the hips up and skimping on the range of motion. Kick the feet all the way forward and all the way back.

BEAR CRAWL

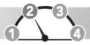

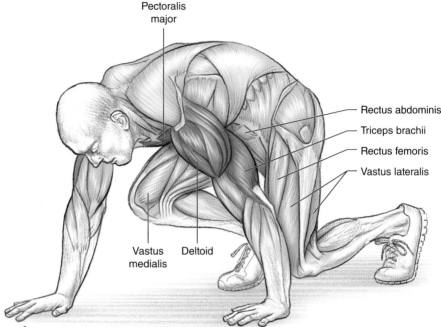

Pectoralis major

Rectus abdominis

Triceps brachii

Rectus femoris

Vastus lateralis

Vastus medialis

Deltoid

Execution

1. Facing downward and keeping your head and neck in neutral alignment, start on all fours so your hands and feet are in contact with the ground.

2. Keeping low to the ground, crawl forward like a bear by flexing the arm and hip on one side of the body while simultaneously extending the arm and hip on the other side of the body.

3. Crawl forward for the desired length and then crawl backward to starting position.

Muscles Involved

Primary: Triceps brachii, pectoralis major, deltoids

Secondary: Hip flexors (iliacus, psoas), quadriceps (rectus femoris, vastus lateralis, vastus medialis, vastus intermedius), rectus abdominis

Exercise Notes

The bear crawl exercise is a natural movement, but your body will want to touch the knees to the ground like you crawled as a baby. Don't allow the knees to touch the ground and avoid looking up and hyperextending the neck. Stay low to the ground and move rhythmically and smoothly. The outside knee of the flexing hip will track on the outside of the adjacent extending arm. Crawling forward will probably seem easy at first, but crawling backward takes practice to develop coordination.

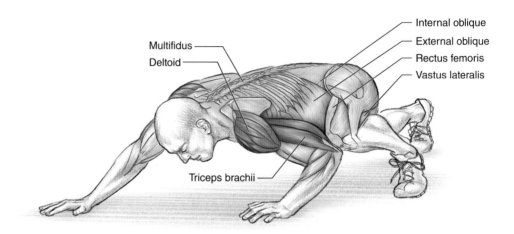

Multifidus

Deltoid

Internal oblique

External oblique

Rectus femoris

Vastus lateralis

Triceps brachii

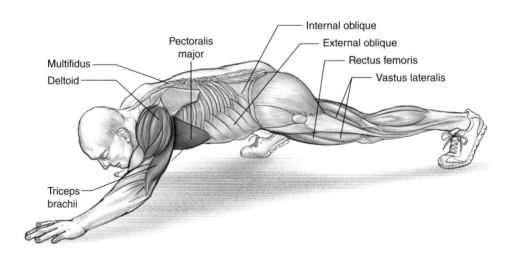

Multifidus

Deltoid

Pectoralis major

Internal oblique

External oblique

Rectus femoris

Vastus lateralis

Triceps brachii

Execution

1. Facing down and keeping your head and neck in neutral alignment, start on all fours with your weight on your hands and feet.

2. Sink the upper body as you would in the bottom of a push-up position, then crawl forward like a crocodile by alternating diagonal patterns of opposite shoulder and hip flexion and shoulder and hip extension combined with torso and hip rotation to allow for increased range of motion. Move forward with the hand and foot on opposite sides.

3. Making sure the knees track on the outside of the adjacent arm, crawl forward for the desired length and then crawl backward to starting position.

Muscles Involved

Primary: Pectoralis major, triceps brachii, deltoids

Secondary: Hip flexors (iliacus, psoas), quadriceps (rectus femoris, vastus lateralis, vastus medialis, vastus intermedius), rectus abdominis, external oblique, internal oblique, multifidus

Exercise Notes

The crocodile crawl is a highly challenging calisthenic movement that requires proper synchronization of the upper body, core, and lower body. Stay low to the ground. Rotate across the spine and hips to allow the hips to flex forward sufficiently while crawling. This exercise requires tremendous upper-body endurance, core stability, and hip mobility.

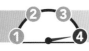
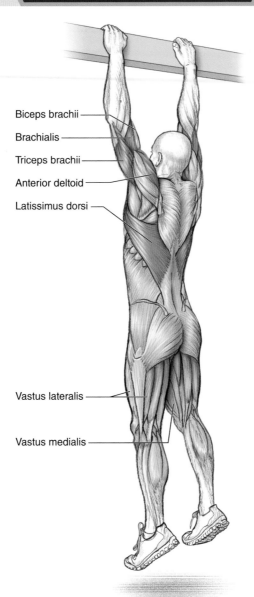

Biceps brachii

Brachialis

Triceps brachii

Anterior deltoid

Latissimus dorsi

Vastus lateralis

Vastus medialis

Execution

1. Stand under a sturdy rafter or chin-up bar. Jump up and grasp the rafter or bar with the hands pronated (palms turned away).

2. Without losing momentum, pull your body up as if performing an explosive pull-up.

3. Keep rising and transition into a dip movement, then lower the body back to starting position.

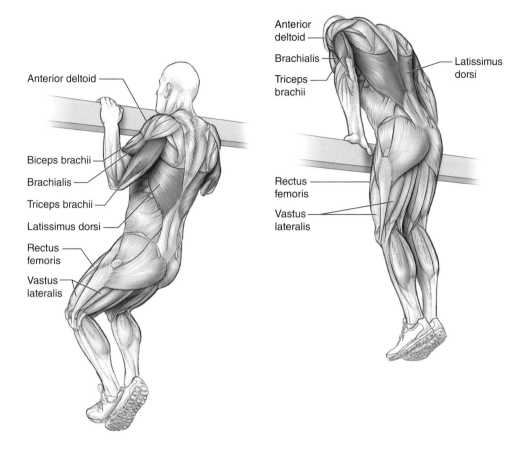

Anterior deltoid

Biceps brachii

Brachialis

Triceps brachii

Latissimus dorsi

Rectus femoris

Vastus lateralis

Anterior deltoid

Brachialis

Triceps brachii

Latissimus dorsi

Rectus femoris

Vastus lateralis

Muscles Involved

Primary: Triceps brachii, pectoralis major, anterior deltoid, latissimus dorsi, brachialis

Secondary: Biceps brachii, quadriceps (rectus femoris, vastus lateralis, vastus medialis, vastus intermedius), rectus abdominis

Exercise Notes

The jumping muscle-up is a highly challenging movement that few people can perform. Before attempting this movement make sure you possess impressive levels of pull-up and dip strength, and even then it will be difficult. You will flow smoothly from a jump to a pull-up to a dip and then reverse the sequence and return to the ground. Incredibly strong people don't require the jumping component. They can perform traditional muscle-ups with no assistance from momentum. The rafter needs to be strong and sturdy to support the exerciser's body weight, and alternatives to a rafter include a chin-up bar or a jungle gym in a local park.

to allow for an accurate estimation. For example, the quality and quantity of sleep you got the night before, how much bad stress (distress) versus good stress (eustress) you have in your life, how motivated you are, and your level of recovery from the week's past workouts can all affect how well you perform in a given training session.

If you're feeling beat up, back off and take it easy for a session or two. If you're extra motivated, feel free to perform an extra set or two. If a certain exercise doesn't feel right, then omit it for the day. Feel free to adjust the intensity, volume, exercise selection, and other variables when you train based on how you feel, but don't feel compelled to stray simply for the sake of straying. It's also perfectly fine to stick to the plan to a T as long as the session feels right.

STRUCTURAL BALANCE

When designing your routine, consider not only the muscles you are working during the session but also the movement patterns you are training. The major muscle groups include the traps, delts, pecs, lats, biceps, triceps, abs, glutes, hams, quads, and calves. You should work all of these muscle groups throughout the week. However, it helps tremendously to think in terms of movement patterns to ensure proper structural balance.

Depending on the classification system, there are six to eight primary movement patterns you should incorporate into each program. For the upper body, you can press and pull in the vertical and horizontal planes. For the lower body, you can perform knee-dominant or hip-dominant exercises. And core training involves linear exercises as well as lateral and rotary exercises. Allow me to elaborate.

A push-up is a horizontal pressing exercise that primarily strengthens the anterior torso musculature. An inverted row is a horizontal pulling exercise that primarily strengthens the posterior torso musculature. If all you ever do are push-ups and you never do inverted rows, you run the risk of developing adducted scapulae and internally rotated shoulders. (Your shoulders would round forward and your arms would turn inward.) Inverted row performance will prevent these negative postural adaptations by strengthening the muscles that counteract these tendencies.

A handstand push-up is a vertical pressing movement while a pull-up is a vertical pulling movement. When executed with proper form in reasonable doses, these exercises work in tandem to create balanced shoulder and scapular (shoulder blade) stability, which helps keep the shoulders healthy.

The squat is a knee-dominant exercise because the knee joint moves through a considerable range of motion, and the quadriceps are taxed heavily. If all you ever do is squat, you'll leave plenty of room on the table for hamstring development, and you could develop knee problems caused by quad dominance, not to mention that you'd lack strength in end-range hip extension.

A reverse hyperextension is a hip-dominant exercise because the movement revolves primarily around the hip joint, with the prime movers being the glutes and hamstrings. The reverse hyper strengthens the posterior chain, which encourages the use of the hamstrings and gluteal musculature while squatting, so you sit back more and rely on the stronger hip muscles to execute the squatting motion. This practice spares the knees and keeps the joints healthy. Synergy exists between the various movement patterns, and balancing these patterns keeps the joints in proper alignment and prevents unnecessary joint stress.

Certain core exercises work primarily in the sagittal plane, which means they produce or prevent movement in linear (front-to-back) patterns. This is in contrast to core exercises that produce or reduce movement in lateral (side-to-side) and rotary (twisting) patterns. Examples of linear core exercises are crunches, sit-ups, and planks. Examples of lateral exercises are partner-assisted oblique raises and side planks. Examples of rotary exercises are windshield wipers and bicycles. It is wise to have a strong core in all directions, so include a balance of linear, lateral, and rotary core exercises.

And last but not least, it's beneficial to incorporate single-limb training into the mix rather than sticking solely to double-limb exercise. Single-limb training works the muscles in a different manner than double-limb exercises. For example, a Bulgarian split squat requires the hip adductors and hip abductors to fire in synchronization in order to stabilize the femur and keep the knee joint tracking properly over the foot. Single-leg stability is critical for optimal performance. To provide another example, a one-arm push-up not only requires considerable pectoral, shoulder, and triceps strength, but also rotary stability throughout the core region to prevent the body from shifting and rotating. For these reasons you should include single-limb training in your program. As you advance, single-limb training becomes critical for bodyweight training because double-limb training won't always provide an adequate challenge.

To reiterate, an ideal routine has a good balance between horizontal pressing and pulling, vertical pressing and pulling, knee-dominant and hip-dominant exercises, linear, lateral, and rotary core exercises, and bilateral (double-limb) and unilateral (single-limb) movements. It is not mandatory to include every pattern in each workout, and it is not mandatory that you perfectly balance the number of sets you perform for opposing movement patterns. Furthermore, it's okay if the majority of your exercises are performed bilaterally. What is important is that you keep in mind the idea of structural balance and avoid skewing your programming toward any particular movement pattern.

Table 11.1 lists all of the exercises in the book and identifies them based on the categories discussed in this section. You will use this chart if you stick with the whole-body routine. If you choose a lower–upper split routine, a push–pull routine, or a body part split routine, you will simply choose exercises according the muscles you are working and won't need to use this table. But it's still a good idea to understand the movement patterns of the exercises rather than just by muscles worked, so I recommend that you pay attention to this chart regardless of the training routine you choose.

Now I'd like to discuss how the nature of your training goals affect your programming.

Table 11.1   Bodyweight Exercises

Exercise	Page number	Exercise level	Horizontal pressing	Horizontal pulling	Vertical pressing	Vertical pulling	Knee dominant	Hip dominant	Linear core	Lateral & rotary core	Targeted movement	Whole body	Bilateral	Unilateral
ARMS														
Triceps extension	8	3									●		●	
Short-lever triceps extension	9	2									●		●	
Short-lever inverted curl	10	2									●		●	
Long-lever inverted curl	11	3									●		●	
Biceps chin-up	12	3				●							●	
Narrow triceps push-up	14	3	●										●	
Diamond triceps push-up	15	3	●										●	
Short-lever triceps push-up	15	2	●										●	
Three-point bench dip	16	2			●								●	
NECK AND SHOULDERS														
Wall anterior neck isohold	22	2									●			
Wall posterior neck isohold	23	2									●			
Manual neck isohold	24	1									●			
Push-back	26	2			●								●	
Feet-elevated pike push-up	28	3			●								●	
Three-point pike push-up	29	4			●								●	
Rear deltoid raise	30	2									●		●	

Exercise	Page number	Exercise level	Horizontal pressing	Horizontal pulling	Vertical pressing	Vertical pulling	Knee dominant	Hip dominant	Linear core	Lateral & rotary core	Targeted movement	Whole body	Bilateral	Unilateral
NECK AND SHOULDERS *(continued)*														
YTWL	32	1									●		●	
Wall handstand push-up	34	4			●								●	
CHEST														
Push-up	38	2	●										●	
Short-lever push-up	39	2	●										●	
Wide-width push-up	39	3	●										●	
Elevated push-up	40	3	●										●	
Short-lever elevated push-up	41	2	●										●	
Torso-elevated push-up	42	1	●										●	
Feet-elevated push-up	43	3	●										●	
Side-to-side push-up	44	3	●											●
Sliding side-to-side push-up	45	3	●											●
One-arm push-up	46	4	●											●
Self-assisted one-arm push-up	47	3	●											●
Clapping push-up	48	3	●										●	
Knee clapping push-up	49	3	●										●	
Whole-body clapping push-up	49	4	●										●	
Chest dip	50	3			●								●	

(continued)

Table 11.1, *continued*

Exercise	Page number	Exercise level	Horizontal pressing	Horizontal pulling	Vertical pressing	Vertical pulling	Knee dominant	Hip dominant	Linear core	Lateral & rotary core	Targeted movement	Whole body	Bilateral	Unilateral
CHEST (continued)														
Sliding fly	52	4									●		●	
Short-lever sliding fly	53	3									●		●	
CORE														
Crunch	60	1							●					
Reverse crunch	61	1							●					
Side crunch	61	1								●				
Superman	62	1							●				●	
Bicycle	63	1								●				●
Seated knee-up	64	1							●				●	
L-sit	65	4							●				●	
Bent-knee single-leg lowering with extension	66	1							●					●
Dead bug	67	2							●					●
Double-leg lowering with bent knees	68	1							●				●	
Lying straight-leg raise	69	2							●				●	
Dragon flag	69	4							●				●	
Bent-leg sit-up	70	1							●					
Straight-leg sit-up	71	1							●					
Twisting sit-up	71	1								●				
Front plank	72	1							●					
Short-lever front plank	73	1							●					

Exercise	Page number	Exercise level	Horizontal pressing	Horizontal pulling	Vertical pressing	Vertical pulling	Knee dominant	Hip dominant	Linear core	Lateral & rotary core	Targeted movement	Whole body	Bilateral	Unilateral
CORE *(continued)*														
Feet-elevated front plank	73	2							●					
Rotating three-point plank	74	2								●				
Rotating two-point plank	75	3								●				
Partner-assisted oblique raise	76	3								●				
RKC plank	77	2							●					
Side plank	78	2								●				
Short-lever side plank	79	1								●				
Feet-elevated side plank	79	3								●				
Hanging leg raise with bent knees	80	2							●				●	
Straight-leg hanging leg raise	81	3							●				●	
Hanging leg raise with reverse crunch	81	3							●				●	
Oblique hanging leg raise	82	3								●			●	
Windshield wiper	83	4								●			●	
Sliding rollout from knees	84	3							●				●	
Standing rollout	85	4							●					
Sliding body saw	86	3							●					

(continued)

Exercise	Page number	Exercise level	Horizontal pressing	Horizontal pulling	Vertical pressing	Vertical pulling	Knee dominant	Hip dominant	Linear core	Lateral & rotary core	Targeted movement	Whole body	Bilateral	Unilateral
BACK														
Pull-up	92	3				●							●	
Rafter pull-up	93	3				●							●	
Side-to-side pull-up	94	4				●								●
Sliding side-to-side pull-up	95	4				●								●
Towel pull-up	96	3				●							●	
One-arm self-assisted chin-up	97	4				●								●
Modified inverted row	98	2		●									●	
Feet-elevated inverted row	99	3		●									●	
Towel inverted row	99	2		●									●	
Side-to-side inverted row	100	4		●										●
Sliding side-to-side inverted row	101	4		●										●
One-arm inverted row	101	4		●										●
Scapular shrug	102	3									●		●	
Corner scapular shrug	103	1												
Towel face pull	104	1		●									●	
THIGHS														
Sumo squat	109	2					●						●	
Wall squat isohold	110	1					●						●	
Wall squat march	111	3					●							●

Exercise	Page number	Exercise level	Horizontal pressing	Horizontal pulling	Vertical pressing	Vertical pulling	Knee dominant	Hip dominant	Linear core	Lateral & rotary core	Targeted movement	Whole body	Bilateral	Unilateral
THIGHS *(continued)*														
Box squat	112	1					●						●	
Low box squat	113	2					●						●	
Jump box squat	113	2					●						●	
Full squat	114	1					●						●	
Counterbalance full squat	115	1					●						●	
Jump full squat	115	2					●						●	
Sissy squat	116	2									●		●	
Single-leg box squat	118	3					●							●
Single-leg low-box squat	119	3					●							●
Jumping single-leg box squat	119	4					●							●
Skater squat	120	3					●							●
Skater squat with knee raise	121	3					●							●
Jumping skater squat	121	3					●							●
Pistol squat	122	4					●							●
Towel pistol squat	123	2					●							●
Static lunge	124	1					●							●
Forward lunge	125	2					●							●
Alternating jump lunge	125	3					●							●
Reverse lunge	126	2					●							●

(continued)

Table 11.1, *continued*

Exercise	Page number	Exercise level	Horizontal pressing	Horizontal pulling	Vertical pressing	Vertical pulling	Knee dominant	Hip dominant	Linear core	Lateral & rotary core	Targeted movement	Whole body	Bilateral	Unilateral
THIGHS (continued)														
Deficit reverse lunge	127	2					●							●
Step-up and reverse lunge hybrid	127	2					●							●
Sliding lunge	128	2					●							●
Step-up	130	1					●							●
High step-up	131	2					●							●
Alternating jump step-up	131	2					●							●
Bulgarian split squat	132	2					●							●
Deficit split squat	133	2					●							●
Jump split squat	133	3					●							●
Russian leg curl	134	3									●		●	
Partner-assisted Russian leg curl	135	3									●		●	
No-hands Russian leg curl	135	4									●		●	
Single-leg Romanian deadlift	136	1						●						●
Reaching Romanian deadlift with knee raise	137	2						●						●
Partner-assisted back extension	138	1						●					●	
Prisoner back extension	139	2						●					●	
Single-leg back extension	139	2						●						●

Exercise	Page number	Exercise level	Horizontal pressing	Horizontal pulling	Vertical pressing	Vertical pulling	Knee dominant	Hip dominant	Linear core	Lateral & rotary core	Targeted movement	Whole body	Bilateral	Unilateral
THIGHS *(continued)*														
Reverse hyper	140	1						●					●	
Single-leg reverse hyper	141	1						●						●
Sliding leg curl	142	3									●		●	
GLUTES														
Glute bridge	146	1						●					●	
Glute march	147	2						●						●
Single-leg glute bridge	147	2						●						●
Shoulder-elevated hip thrust	148	1						●					●	
Shoulder-elevated hip thrust march	149	2						●						●
Single-leg hip thrust	149	2						●						●
Shoulder-and-feet-elevated hip thrust	150	2						●					●	
Single-leg shoulder-and-feet-elevated hip thrust	151	4						●						●
Donkey kick	152	1						●						●
Bent-leg donkey kick	153	1						●						●
Bird dog	153	1						●						●
Side-lying clam	154	1									●			●
Side-lying clam at neutral position	155	1									●			●
Side-lying hip raise	156	3									●			●

(continued)

Table 11.1, *continued*

Exercise	Page number	Exercise level	Horizontal pressing	Horizontal pulling	Vertical pressing	Vertical pulling	Knee dominant	Hip dominant	Linear core	Lateral & rotary core	Targeted movement	Whole body	Bilateral	Unilateral
CALVES														
Elevated calf raise	160	1									●		●	
Single-leg elevated calf raise	161	1									●			●
Squat calf raise	162	1									●		●	
Stiff-leg ankle hop	164	2									●		●	
Single-leg ankle hop	165	2									●			●
WHOLE BODY														
Jumping jack	170	1										●	●	
Transverse-arm jumping jack	171	1										●	●	
Burpee	172	2										●	●	
Burpee with push-up, jump, and reach	173	3										●	●	
Push-up with hip extension	174	2										●	●	
Towel row isohold with glute march	176	3										●	●	
Sit-up to stand with jump and reach	178	3										●	●	
Mountain climber	180	3										●		●
Bear crawl	181	2										●		●
Crocodile crawl	182	3										●		●
Jumping muscle-up	184	4										●	●	
Crab walk	186	2										●		●

TRAINING GOALS

People choose to exercise for many reasons. Some want to improve their general health, some want to build larger muscles, some want to shed fat, some seek to get stronger, some hope to improve their functional strength and athleticism, and some strive to eliminate joint dysfunction and prevent injury. Bodybuilders seek maximum hypertrophy (muscularity), powerlifters seek maximum strength, weightlifters seek maximum power, and sprinters seek maximum speed. It should come as no surprise that their training methods differ substantially because training for a particular purpose affects the way a person trains.

Sport-Specific Training

In general, there is too much hype surrounding the topic of sport-specific training. While it is true that athletes from different sports require unique types of strength and energy system development, ideally every athlete should display sound movement patterns and athleticism. This is why it's essential to master the basics as you lay the foundation for subsequent adaptations. You want to make sure that you analyze your sport and perform exercises that use the same muscles and mimic the movement patterns and directions found in the sport, but don't get too carried away to the point that you lose sight of the basics. All athletes should possess balanced strength and mobility. Single-leg exercises such as Bulgarian split squats and single-leg hip thrusts and core-stability exercises such as RKC planks and side planks are great exercises for all athletes.

Strength

When you train for maximal strength you want to perform multijoint movements, stay in lower repetition ranges, and rest more between sets. With bodyweight training, this is not always feasible. For example, the squat, bench press, and deadlift are three of the most popular exercises in resistance training because they use a lot of muscles and allow you to lift large loads. However, in bodyweight training, although you can tweak exercises to make them easier or more challenging according to your level of strength, the most resistance you'll ever use is equal to your body weight. For this reason it can be difficult to develop maximal strength solely through bodyweight training.

The best approach to developing maximal strength through bodyweight training is to lay down an excellent foundation of flexibility, stability, and motor control. This provides a base for future gains and advancement to more challenging exercise variations. I read an interview with a U.S. Olympic gymnastics coach who said that although his gymnasts never performed resistance training and solely performed bodyweight exercises, many of them could bench press double their bodyweight and deadlift triple their bodyweight. Clearly a person who performs advanced variations of bodyweight exercises can develop impressive levels of strength. Master the basics and then progress to single-limb exercises, plyometrics, and other advanced methods.

Hypertrophy

When training for maximum muscularity make sure you add sets of higher repetitions and training that targets certain regions of the body, along with resting less between sets. While strength is paramount for hypertrophy, the relationship isn't linear. Always feel the intended muscles working and use controlled form through a full range of motion. A variety of repetition ranges is ideal for muscle growth as is a large variety of exercises to stimulate all of the regions of the muscles.

Body Part Specialization

Sometimes you'll want to focus on bringing up a particular area of the body, perhaps the delts, glutes, upper pecs, or lats. In this case you simply need to cut back slightly on work for the rest of the body while adding work for the weaker muscle group. Other times you may want to improve a particular skill. For example, you might want to be able to perform a one-arm push-up or a pistol squat. In this case you can train the skill frequently while scaling back the rest of your routine. You can't continuously add to your programs. When you add something, you have to take something out or you run the risk of overdoing it and stagnating or worse, regressing.

Let's say that you can't perform a chin-up. Rather than just performing back exercises a couple of times per week in your regular program, you could choose to perform two sets of negative chin-ups several times each day. When you are relatively weak, you don't stress the body as much when exercising, so the added frequency will expedite your progress and allow you to perform regular chin-ups in much less time. But stick to just one movement or one body part at a time. If you try to pick two movements or two body parts, it's no longer a specialization routine. You're just getting greedy. Don't go overboard or you'll pay the price by stagnating.

Fat Loss

When focusing on weight loss, retain as much muscle as possible to ensure that the pounds shed are composed of fat rather than muscle mass. This is the key to a quality physique. Remember that what builds muscle keeps muscle, so your training doesn't have to change much. Train for strength and simply add a couple of MRT circuits or HIIT sessions (see chapter 10) during your training week and focus on your diet. I'll expound on this later in this chapter.

Now it's time to tell you about acute training variables in strength training.

TRAINING VARIABLES

You should understand 10 common training variables in strength and conditioning. I'll briefly touch on each of them.

Exercise Selection

This appears to be a simple category, but it's probably the most poorly understood training variable in the world. Folks don't seem to want to stick to exercises within their current level of ability. When you go to the gym and see people's hips sagging during push-ups, bodies flailing during chin-ups, backs rounding during deadlifts, and bars rebounding off of chests during bench presses, you quickly realize that most people have a compelling need to feel strong and athletic. Unfortunately, they're doing more harm than good by using too much weight or performing exercises too advanced for their abilities.

It is imperative that you understand regressions and progressions. For example, a box squat is easier than a full squat, a static lunge is easier than a pistol squat, and a knee push-up is easier than a feet-elevated push-up. Stick with the proper exercise variation for your current level of ability, and once you've mastered it, progress to a more challenging exercise. If you can't perform a particular exercise properly, find a way to make it easier so you can perform it properly. By regressing to a simpler variation, you'll develop sound motor patterns that will allow you to progress more rapidly.

Consider structural balance when you choose your exercises, and vary the exercises over time to reduce the risk of habituation and pattern overload. You'll always perform the same basic movement patterns, but the exercises will differ to provide the novel training stimulus needed for continuous positive adaptation.

Exercise Order

The exercises you perform first in the routine will produce the best stimuli and respond best to your training. If you seek improvements on chin-ups, perform them first in your sessions. If your goal is to raise your pistol squat from 3 to 10 repetitions, place them first in the workout. Whatever it is that you're trying to improve most, prioritize it in your programming.

Alternate between agonistic and antagonistic movements, opposing motions such as pushing and pulling in the horizontal plane, in your training sessions. This gives your body natural rest periods. For example, you can perform a set of push-ups, then a set of inverted rows, then a set of push-ups, and so forth. This is called antagonistic pairing, and it allows you to keep your metabolism revved while providing increased rest time for the working muscles. The key is to select movements that don't interfere with each other and that use opposing patterns. Don't choose push-ups and handstand push-ups for pairing because they train many of the same muscles.

In general, the largest muscle groups should be trained first and the smallest should be trained last, unless you are specializing in a particular body part. A broad rule of thumb is to perform knee-dominant exercises (quads) first, then hip-dominant exercises (hamstrings and glutes), then upper-body pulls (back), then upper-body presses (chest and shoulders), and then smaller muscles such as core and targeted exercises (abs, obliques, biceps, triceps).

If performing power training, strength training, and conditioning in the same session, perform them in that order. Train power when you're fresh, strength in the middle, and conditioning last.

Split

Your training split refers to how you split up your workouts throughout the week. Several types of popular training splits exist. The most common are whole-body training, lower–upper splits, push–pull routines, and body part splits.

During whole-body training, you work the entire body each session, so technically you're not splitting anything up. This approach is wisest for bodyweight training. In lower–upper splits you work half of the body in one session and the other half of the body in the next session. For example, you work legs one session and upper body the next. Push–pull routines alternate between sessions that work the pushing muscles (quads, chest, shoulders, triceps) with sessions that work the pulling muscles (hamstrings, back, biceps). Body part splits focus on one or two body parts each session, for example, chest and triceps, back and biceps, legs, or shoulders and traps.

Bodybuilders tend to stick to body part splits. Powerlifters tend to stick to lower–upper splits. Olympic lifters and strongmen tend to stick to whole-body training. People who perform solely bodyweight training are drawn toward whole-body training and they develop amazing physiques, as do gymnasts. When you examine the routines of people who are achieving the best possible physiques with bodyweight training, you realize that most are performing whole-body routines.

Frequency

Training frequency refers to the number of days per week you train. Typically exercisers train two to six days per week; three to five days is the most common. The number of days you train depends on your personal situation, but I recommend choosing frequency over volume, which I'll explain next. It's more fruitful to train four days per week for 30 minutes a session than to train two days per week for 60 minutes a session. Whatever you choose, make sure you train the entire body each week.

Volume

Strength trainers argue over ideal volume. Some believe that low volume is ideal, while most others believe that higher volume is better. Usually the truth lies somewhere in the middle.

Volume generally refers to the number of sets and repetitions you perform. For example, a low-volume session could include one set of six exercises, whereas a high-volume session could include three sets of eight exercises.

Most strength trainers agree that no matter how many sets you perform, the first set is by far the most important, and subsequent sets become less important. The law of diminishing returns applies to programming. For example, performing 1 set of push-ups is good, performing 3 sets is even better, but performing 20 sets is not ideal. There comes a point at which additional sets become counterproductive because the muscles aren't able to repair themselves for future sessions.

Of course, form and intensity are factors here. The lifter who has crummy form can't handle much volume, and the lifter who doesn't push the intensity envelope very far can handle plenty of volume. Volume and intensity are inversely related. You can train hard or you can train long but you can't do both.

Furthermore, the type of split influences volume considerations. A lifter performing whole-body routines needs his or her muscles to be fresh for the following workout, but a lifter adhering to a body part split typically has more time to recover because this lifter usually hits a particular body part just once or twice per week.

Intensity

Intensity usually refers to the amount of weight you lift. This is more applicable to resistance training when you're using barbell and dumbbell loads, but it applies to bodyweight training as well. Intensity can refer to intensity of load, and certain exercises involve more load than others. For example, a push-up involves about 68 percent of one's body weight, not 100 percent, because there are several points of support and the body is at an angle at the top of the movement. Elevating the feet increases the percentage of body weight in the push-up, and performing a one-arm push-up dramatically increases the loading on the shoulder joint. As you progress to more challenge exercises, your exercise intensity increases in terms of joint loading.

Intensiveness

In comparison to intensity, intensiveness is sometimes referred to as intensity of effort. Many people believe that the terms *intensity* and *intensiveness* are interchangeable, but intensity refers to the load used and the other refers to the effort put forth. Intensiveness is simply how hard you push yourself during the session. Some days you'll feel great and push it at 95 percent. Other days you'll strive for 70 percent. If you push too hard for too long, you'll spin your wheels by overreaching, and, even worse, you could enter the tumultuous waters of overtraining. The body has a natural way of asking you to back off, and it's important to listen to biofeedback and pay attention to these signals.

Density

Dense materials are packed closely together, whereas loose materials are not. Similarly, dense workouts are packed with activity. Training density generally refers to the amount of work you do per session. If you perform a 60-minute workout but rest 5 minutes between each set, you end up performing just eight sets, and your workout is not very dense. Conversely, if you perform 25 sets in 60 minutes, your session is quite dense. There's an optimal balance because strength training is not supposed to mimic aerobic exercise. You should push hard and then rest between sets, but don't rest too long.

More challenging exercises such as Bulgarian split squats and chin-ups require more rest between sets, whereas simpler exercises such as crunches and bird dogs do not require much rest. Antagonistic pairing is a way to increase training density, but don't get too hung up on this category. The exerciser who does circuit training but fails to get stronger over time doesn't realize nearly as much gain as the exerciser who dramatically increases his or her strength, even if the training isn't very dense. Some exercises don't require rest between sets, while others do. Most of the time, aim for 30 to 90 seconds of rest between sets.

Tempo

Tempo is an interesting variable to tinker with because bodyweight training lends itself to tempo alterations. Tempo is usually indicated with three numbers. The first number refers to the concentric (muscles shorten during contraction) portion of the repetition, the second number to the isometric (lockout) portion of the movement, and the third number to the eccentric (muscles lengthen during contraction) portion. So a 1-0-3 tempo requires an exerciser to lift the body weight in one second and then lower the body in three seconds for each repetition. A 2-3-5 tempo calls for two seconds concentric, three seconds of isometric pause at the top, and five seconds of eccentric for each repetition.

An isohold involves holding a movement in a static position for time. You can hold the bottom position of a push-up or static lunge to build mobility and stability in those positions. You can also hold the top of a chin-up or single-leg hip thrust to build strength and stability in those positions.

A pause repetition requires you to pause briefly (usually one to five seconds) at a certain position in the exercise, for example the bottom of a push-up or Bulgarian split squat or the top of an inverted row or hip thrust.

Negative-accentuated repetitions are performed by slowly and gradually lowering yourself eccentrically. For example, you could lower yourself in a chin-up or dip exercise for a count of 10 seconds.

Explosive repetitions are performed with maximal acceleration, which can vary depending on the goal. For example, if trying to hone in on the pectorals during push-ups, you can descend rapidly and quickly reverse the movement. If trying to focus on triceps power, you can perform a plyometric push-up and explode off the ground and then catch yourself in the upper range of the movement.

Partial repetitions can be done successfully from time to time to provide a novel training stimulus. Full repetitions are better for strength and hypertrophy but sometimes it's wise to perform partials. For example, during push-ups or dips you may choose to focus on the bottom range of motion and avoid going all the way up as a strategy to target the pectorals. Or you may decide to perform as many full-range repetitions as possible and then switch to partials to continue the set and increase the set's intensiveness.

Provide variety in bodyweight training by manipulating the tempo and using unique repetition strategies.

Periodization

Entire books have been written on the topic of periodization, so I'll try to be brief. Periodization simply refers to how you switch up your workouts over time. Lifters who have a goal and a plan see much better results than those who waltz into the gym aimlessly and just fool around.

You can periodize your workouts in an infinite number of ways. For example, one month you perform higher repetitions, the next month medium repetitions, and the following month lower repetitions. Or, maybe one month you incorporate isoholds, the next you accentuate the negative portion of certain exercises, and the following month you incorporate plyometric exercises. You could focus on core strength for two weeks, then upper-body strength for two weeks, and then lower-body strength for two weeks. These are just a few periodization strategies.

Simply progressing to more challenging exercise variations over time is also a method of periodization. Coaches sometimes plan entire years of training for their athletes, but for most exercisers this is unnecessary because you can achieve excellent results by having a general plan and simply training according to feel. What's most important is that you progress in your workouts by using better form, performing more repetitions, and increasing intensity, intensiveness, and density.

I am now going to teach you how to put it all together by providing sample routines.

PUTTING IT ALL TOGETHER

There are numerous ways to put together a successful routine, and no single program is best for everyone. What works for one person might not work for another, and what works for you this month might not work for you six months from now. That said, some programs are much better than others. I've equipped you with sound information on program design. You've learned the basics and have a good head start. If you're a beginner, stick to one of the routines I've provided. But as you advance, adapt these programs to better suit your preference and physiology.

With bodyweight exercises, it's difficult to recommend repetition ranges because they vary according to your level of strength and conditioning. For example, three sets of 15 repetitions for the push-up exercise will be too challenging for many people and too easy for others. For this reason I include only the number of sets next to the exercises.

The programs are written in template style so you can learn the patterns of well-planned workouts and substitute exercises according to your current level of fitness. Categories of exercises designated as A1 and A2, B1 and B2, and so on, indicate paired supersets in which you perform one exercise after the other with no rest between. Perform a set of exercise number one then a set of exercise number two. Rest a minute, then go back to exercise one, and so forth until you have performed the prescribed number of sets.

I've included a template for a whole-body routine, a lower–upper split routine, a push–pull routine, and a body part split routine.

Whole-Body Routine

Perform the routine in table 11.2 two to five times per week. Vary the movements throughout the week. This is the style of training that I recommend to exercisers sticking to bodyweight training. This routine includes paired supersets, and the targeted exercises at the end of the workout provide you an opportunity to target specific muscles but prevent you from overdoing it with too much volume.

Table 11.2   Sample Whole-Body Routine

	Type of exercise	Sample exercises	Number of sets
A1	Knee dominant	Box squat (beginner) or pistol squat (advanced)	3
A2	Upper-body pulling	Modified inverted row (intermediate) or side-to-side pull-up (advanced)	3
B1	Hip dominant	Single-leg Romanian deadlift (beginner) or single-leg hip thrust (intermediate)	3
B2	Upper-body pressing	Torso-elevated push-up (beginner) or one-arm push-up (advanced)	3
C1	Linear core	Crunch (beginner) or hanging leg raise with bent knees (intermediate)	1
C2	Lateral and rotary core	Side crunch (beginner) or side plank (intermediate)	1
D1	Targeted movement	Towel rear deltoid raise (intermediate) or sliding fly (advanced)	1
D2	Targeted movement	Elevated calf raise (beginner) or scapular shrug (intermediate–advanced)	1

Lower–Upper Split Routine

Perform two lower-body and two upper-body sessions each week. Perform all exercises (table 11.3) in straight-set fashion: Execute each set consecutively for a particular exercise before moving on to the next exercise.

Table 11.3   Sample Lower–Upper Split Routine

	Type of exercise	Sample exercises	Number of sets
		DAY 1 AND DAY 3: LOWER BODY	
1	Quad	Full squat (beginner) or Bulgarian split squat (intermediate)	3
2	Hamstring	Reverse hyper (beginner) or no-hands Russian leg curl (advanced)	3
3	Glute	Glute bridge (beginner) or shoulder-elevated hip thrust march (intermediate)	3
4	Ab superset	Bent-leg sit-up (beginner) and side plank (intermediate) or sliding rollout from knees (intermediate–advanced) and windshield wiper (advanced)	2
		DAY 2 AND DAY 4: UPPER BODY	
1	Pec	Torso-elevated push-up (beginner) or clapping push-up (intermediate–advanced)	3
2	Back	Towel face pull (beginner) or sliding side-to-side pull-up (advanced)	3
3	Shoulder	Push back (intermediate) or feet elevated pike push-up (intermediate–advanced)	2
4	Arm superset	Short-lever inverted curl (intermediate) and short-lever triceps extension (intermediate) or rafter biceps chin-up (intermediate–advanced) and diamond triceps push-up (intermediate–advanced)	2

Push–Pull Routine

Perform two push sessions and two pull sessions each week. See table 11.4.

Table 11.4   Sample Push–Pull Routine

	Type of exercise	Sample exercises	Number of sets
		DAY 1 AND DAY 3: PUSHING	
A1	Quad	Sumo squat (beginner) or high step-up (intermediate)	3
A2	Upper-body pressing	Short-lever elevated push-up (intermediate) or wall handstand push-up (advanced)	3
B1	Glute	Glute bridge (beginner) or single-leg hip thrust (intermediate)	3
B2	Triceps	Short-lever triceps push-up (intermediate) or three-point bench dip (intermediate)	2
C	Ab	Lying straight-leg raise (intermediate) or L-sit (advanced)	2

(continued)

Table 11.4   Sample Push–Pull Routine *(continued)*

	Type of exercise	Sample exercises	Number of sets
		DAY TWO AND DAY FOUR: PULLING	
A1	Hamstring	Partner-assisted back extension (beginner) or sliding leg curl (intermediate–advanced)	3
A2	Upper-body pulling	Modified inverted row (intermediate) or sliding side-to-side inverted row (advanced)	3
B1	Additional pulling movement for back or hamstrings	Reaching Romanian deadlift with knee raise (intermediate) or one-arm inverted row (advanced)	3
B2	Biceps	Short-lever inverted curl (intermediate) or inverted curl (intermediate–advanced)	2
C	Ab	Bicycle (beginner) or dragon flag (advanced)	2

Body Part Split Routine

Split the sessions so that you train the entire body over three to five days. See table 11.5.

Table 11.5   Sample Body Part Split Routine

	Type of exercise	Sample exercises	Number of sets
		DAY 1: QUADS, GLUTES, ABS	
1	Quad	Reverse lunge (intermediate) or skater squat (intermediate–advanced)	3
2	Upper-body pressing	Wall squat isohold (beginner) or step-up and reverse lunge hybrid (intermediate)	3
3	Glute	Side-lying clam (beginner) or side-lying hip raise (intermediate–advanced)	3
4	Triceps	Reverse crunch (beginner) or rotating two-point plank (intermediate–advanced)	2
5	Ab	Side plank (intermediate) or partner-assisted oblique raise (intermediate–advanced)	2

	Type of exercise	Sample exercises	Number of sets
DAY 2: PECS, SHOULDERS, TRICEPS			
1	Pec	Torso-elevated push-up (beginner) or elevated push-up (intermediate–advanced)	3
2	Pec	Short-lever push-up (intermediate) or sliding fly (advanced)	3
3	Shoulder	Feet-elevated pike push-up (intermediate–advanced) or wall handstand push-up (advanced)	3
4	Shoulder	Push back (intermediate) or rear deltoid raise (intermediate)	2
5	Triceps	Triceps extension (intermediate–advanced) or narrow triceps push-up (intermediate–advanced)	2
DAY 3: HAMS, GLUTES, CALVES			
1	Hamstring	Reverse hyper (beginner) or no-hands Russian leg curl (advanced)	3
2	Hamstring	Reaching Romanian deadlift with knee raise (intermediate) or single-leg back extension (intermediate)	3
3	Glute	Bent-leg donkey kick (beginner) or single-leg shoulder-and-feet-elevated hip thrust (advanced)	3
4	Calf	Elevated calf raise (beginner) or single-leg elevated calf raise (beginner)	2
5	Calf	Squat calf raise (beginner) or single-leg ankle hop (intermediate)	2
DAY 4: BACK, NECK, BICEPS			
1	Back	Towel pull-up (intermediate–advanced) or sliding side-to-side pull-up (advanced)	3
2	Back	Modified inverted row (intermediate) or sliding side-to-side inverted row (advanced)	3
3	Back	Towel face pull (beginner) or scapular shrug (intermediate–advanced)	3
4	Neck	Manual neck isohold (beginner) or wall posterior neck iso-hold (intermediate)	2
5	Biceps	Short-lever inverted curl (intermediate) or long-lever inverted curl (intermediate–advanced)	2

TRAINING FOR FAT LOSS

In the last chapter I discussed HIIT and MRT for fat-loss training. These methods can help you accelerate your fat loss. However, you must remember that when you train hard, you get hungrier. Most people fail in their fat-loss endeavors because even though they train hard, they fail to achieve a caloric deficit. You need to consume fewer calories than you expend if you want to lose weight. Strength training, HIIT, and MRT will cause you to burn more calories and lose weight, but only if you avoid the temptation (especially late at night) to raid the fridge. You will become hungry as you lose weight because your body and hunger hormones seem to want to prevent you from achieving your goals.

You will achieve your optimal physique not through starvation and excessive cardio, but through an intelligent combination of dietary, strength training, and HIIT or MRT practices. Here are some rules of thumb to remember:

- Consume the appropriate number of calories. Most people underestimate the number of calories they consume each day. Many good calorie estimators can easily be found online.

- Consume the ideal proportions of carbohydrate, protein, and health fats. Many people consume too much carbohydrate and not enough protein and healthy fats.

- Prioritize strength training. This is what builds or holds on to muscle tissue so that you burn more fat for weight loss. Avoid the dreaded skinny-fat appearance (someone of normal weight but still carrying extra fat and too little muscle) and instead get and stay strong. Perform three to five strength training sessions per week.

- Add several brief HIIT or MRT sessions per week but don't let these workouts make you so sore that it interferes with the quality of your strength sessions.

You can conduct HIIT workouts on a track or field, in water, on a treadmill, on a bicycle, on a rowing machine, on an elliptical or stair stepper, or other places. Here are sample HIIT and MRT sessions:

Sample HIIT Sessions

HIIT protocol 1: Sprint 10 seconds, walk 50 seconds, perform 10 times. Total workout time is 10 minutes.

HIIT protocol 2: Sprint 30 seconds, walk 90 seconds, perform eight times. Total workout time is 16 minutes.

HIIT protocol 3: Sprint 60 seconds, walk 240 seconds, perform four times. Total workout time is 20 minutes.

Sample MRT Sessions

MRT protocol 1: Choose a knee-dominant lower-body exercise such as a squat and an upper-body pressing exercise such as a push-up. Perform 60 seconds of one exercise, immediately perform 60 seconds of the next exercise, and then rest for 60 seconds. Repeat three times. Now choose a hip-dominant lower-body exercise such as a shoulder-elevated hip thrust and an upper-body pulling exercise such as an inverted row. Perform 60 seconds of one exercise, immediately perform 60 seconds of the next exercise, and then rest for 60 seconds. Perform three times. Total workout time is 18 minutes.

MRT protocol 2: Choose three whole-body exercises from chapter 10. Make sure they differ significantly from each other, for example, burpee, mountain climber, and bear crawl. Perform 30 seconds of one exercise, rest 15 seconds, perform 30 seconds of the second exercise, rest 15 seconds, perform 30 seconds of the third exercise, and then rest 15 seconds. Perform three times. Total workout time is 6 minutes, 45 seconds.

MRT protocol 3: Choose a compound lower-body exercise such as a jump full squat or reverse lunge, a compound upper-body exercise such as a pike push-up or a chin-up, and a whole-body exercise such as a push-up with hip extension or a towel row isohold with glute march. Perform 30 seconds of one exercise, rest 15 seconds, perform 30 seconds of the second exercise, rest 15 seconds, perform 30 seconds of the third exercise, and then rest 15 seconds. Perform three times. Total workout time is 6 minutes, 45 seconds.

As I stated previously, there are plenty of ways to create an effective HIIT or MRT session, so feel free to tinker with the work times, rest times, and total times.

ABOUT THE AUTHOR

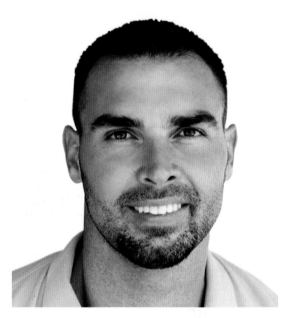

Bret Contreras, MS, CSCS, has become known in the strength and conditioning industry as The Glute Guy because of his expertise in helping clients develop strong, shapely glutes. He is currently pursuing a PhD in sport science at the Auckland University of Technology in New Zealand, where he has studied under biomechanics expert John Cronin. Contreras has conducted numerous electromyography experiments in his research.

As the former owner of Lifts Studio in Scottsdale, Arizona, Contreras worked closely with hundreds of clients ranging from sedentary people to elite athletes, and he invented a glute-strengthening machine called the Skorcher. He currently trains figure competitors, writes programs for clients from all over the world, and consults for various professional sport teams.

Contreras is a distinguished lecturer in strength and conditioning, presenting at many conferences throughout the United States, including the 2013 NSCA Personal Trainer Conference. He is a peer-reviewed author and regular contributor to well-known industry publications including *Men's Health, Men's Fitness, Oxygen,* and *MuscleMag. Oxygen* magazine voted him the Glute Expert in their 2010 glutes edition. Contreras maintains The Strength of Evidence Podcast, where he discusses important topics in strength and conditioning, and a popular blog at www.BretContreras.com.